TOO SWEET

The not-so-serious side to diabetes

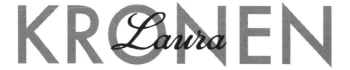

KRONEN

Laura

Be You Only Better Books

Copyright © 2014 Laura Kronen

Cover photo by Kelly Wachs

ISBN: 1495452050
ISBN 13: 9781495452055

Library of Congress Control Number: 2014902503
CreateSpace Independent Publishing Platform
North Charleston, South Carolina

For my type 3 diabetics...

I love you more than anything

Contents

How to Use This Book

Start here, at the beginning, read all of the words one after the other until you come to the very end, and then stop. Do not take this too seriously. Don't make any changes to your personal diabetes management or to someone else's. Do not adjust your treatment or the treatment of others without consulting a doctor. I am not a doctor, nor do I play one on television. It has never crossed my mind to go to medical school, and I am not qualified in any way whatsoever to give medical advice. I've never dated a doctor, and none of my siblings or immediate family members are doctors, although I admit I *do* have one superstar second cousin who is a brain surgeon. What I am, however, is a diabetic person. I have type 1 diabetes, I have lived with it for the past twenty years, and I have a lot to say about the subject.

Consider me someone with whom you can easily talk and with whom you can share adventures, cocktails, and the same fabulous disease. Laugh and commiserate with me as we go through all aspects of living with an ailment that is chock full of so many variables. Diabetes is definitely not cookie-cutter; no two people can sit down and eat Double Stuff Oreos and each require the same amount of insulin, even if those two people are the same height and weight and are just as good looking. Managing diabetes is not a science, it is an art.

The purpose of this book is to entertain, not to change the way you, or anyone you know, does business with diabetes. Again, please do not make any alterations to your treatment plan based upon what you read here without discussing them with your doctor. Have I said that enough? Now that we've got that settled, kick back and enjoy this sugary delight. I promise it won't raise your blood glucose level.

Why I Wrote This Book

Why am I wide awake? I pick up my iPhone, which also conveniently acts as my nightlight, and check the time—3:12 AM. I'm feeling very warm, although I know I have the air turned down to the perfect sleeping temperature of sixty-nine degrees. This can only mean one thing. I check my blood. Coincidentally, it reads 312, the same as the time. Although my blood sugar is crazy high, the irony amuses me ever so slightly. Then my symptoms come alive. As I blink, my eyelids make a clicking noise, my heart is racing, and my brain is in a fog. My fingers feel stiff, which in my head I have associated with the high levels of sugar in my blood crystallizing together. Not sure if there is any truth to that, but this book is not entirely based upon fact. It is merely a collage of my personal experiences and the experiences of other diabetic people around me. It is a combination of anecdotes and comedic situations, crazy theories, modern-day references, pancreas jokes, and real-life diabetes all rolled into one.

Diabetes isn't funny. Certainly a lot of seriousness goes along with having it. A plethora of somber diabetes-related information is available out there, but you need to balance out all the doom and gloom. The human condition lends itself to humorous situations, and research shows the health advantages of laughter. A humor filter can protect the mind, promote learning, reduce stress, and allow for a processing of emotions in a healthy way.

Either you or someone you know is stuck with this disease, so we might as well make the best of it.

Chapter One

Just the Facts, Ma'am

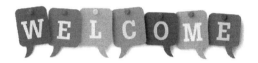

elcome to the diabetics' club. Congratulations! You have an irrevocable, non-
transferable lifetime membership. Whether you,
your child, a friend, or significant other is afflicted,
this disorder is a part of your life forever.

When you have diabetes (and it is *not*
pronounced di-ah-bee-tis like the old guy on
the commercial repeatedly says), it can be hard
to find something to laugh about. The need to
monitor glucose levels, count carbohydrates,
watch your diet, exercise, take pills and inject
insulin—plus the worry about long-term
complications—make diabetes a very serious

and, at times, overwhelming disease. Laughter and a positive attitude are good medicine and have been scientifically proven to benefit your health. Finding the humor in your diabetes can help you endure and make those overwhelming tasks feel more manageable.

Although it seems very basic, let's get some rudimentary facts out of the way before we deal with the crux, the core, the nitty-gritty, and the *reality* of what living with diabetes every day is *really* like.

Diabetes was one of the first-known diseases described in the history of humankind. It's amazing when you think about how long it has been around; it was first described on an Egyptian manuscript circa 1500 BCE as "too great emptying of the urine." Indian physicians around the same time identified the disease as "honey urine," noting that the urine on the ground would attract ants. Back in the dark era of human hygiene, the science of sanitary engineering was apparently very primitive, and open defecation was the way to go.

There are three main types of diabetes: type 1, type 2, and for the sake of all the moms out there we will touch on gestational diabetes as well. No version of the disease is a Sunday afternoon walk in the park. In all cases, your brain now serves as your pancreas, and you have to think about how every morsel of food you put in your mouth will ultimately affect your blood sugar.

Type 1 Diabetes (formerly known as juvenile diabetes)

In this autoimmune disease, a person's pancreas stops producing insulin. It usually strikes in childhood, but the fun can begin at any age and then lasts a lifetime, making it necessary for those with type 1 to inject insulin multiple times daily or to continually infuse through a pump. Although 85 percent of those living with type 1 diabetes are adults, but between 2001 and 2009 there was a 23 percent increase in type 1 among people younger than age twenty. There are currently about three million of us worldwide; to put that into perspective, imagine every person currently living in the state of Mississippi having type 1 diabetes. Coincidentally, Mississippi is also the state currently hosting the greatest percentage of adults diagnosed with diabetes. I know you are now wondering which state has the least. It's Vermont.

Insulin is a hormone produced by special cells in the pancreas called *beta cells*. Insulin is needed to move blood sugar (glucose) into cells, where it is stored and used for energy. In type 1 diabetes, beta cells produce little or no insulin. Without insulin, glucose builds up in the bloodstream instead of going into the cells, and the body is unable to use this glucose for energy. The exact cause of type 1 diabetes is not fully understood. Most likely it is caused by an infection, virus (I'm convinced that's how I got it) or some other trigger that causes the body to mistakenly attack the cells in the pancreas that produce insulin.

Those with type 1 diabetes must check their blood sugar by pricking their finger for blood testing many times a day. While trying to balance insulin doses with their food intake and daily activities, people with this form of diabetes may also experience *hypoglycemia* (low blood sugar) and *hyperglycemia* (high blood sugar), both of which can be life altering and life threatening. I'm not going to mince words here: both conditions suck.

Although insulin injections allow a person with type 1 to stay alive, they do not cure diabetes, and they don't necessarily prevent the disease's devastating side effects (which shall remain nameless, for the sake of our lighthearted and bubbly spin on the subject). Lethal adjectives such as *life-threatening* and *devastating* (and even the word *lethal*) will be kept to a minimum here. The fact is that good control can prevent or delay these complications. This book is an uplifting, cheeky, and sprightly look into the life of someone just like yourself. We are keeping it happy-go-lucky, and this chapter is about as serious as it's going to get.

Type 2 Diabetes (formerly known as adult-onset diabetes)

In type 2 diabetes, a person's body still produces insulin but cannot use it effectively. It is often diagnosed in adulthood but does not usually require injections. Increased obesity has led to a recent rise in cases of type 2 in children and adults. Many times those with type 2 can rid themselves of the disease if they lose weight and maintain a healthy diet. Lucky them! However, it doesn't always work that way.

When you have type 2 diabetes, your fat, liver, and muscle cells do not respond correctly to insulin. This is called *insulin resistance.* As a result, blood sugar is not stored in these cells to be used for energy, and high levels of sugar build up in the blood causing hyperglycemia.

Unlike type 1, which is an autoimmune disorder, type 2 diabetes is a metabolic disorder and usually occurs slowly over time. Many people with the disease are overweight when they are diagnosed. Increased fat makes it harder for the body to use insulin correctly. Sadly, even overweight toddlers are now being diagnosed with type 2 diabetes. This is not to say that type 2 cannot also develop in people who are thin—it can—but this is more common in the elderly.

Family history and genes play the largest role in type 2 diabetes. Low activity level, poor diet, and excess body weight around the waist increase the risk of developing it—and scads of other diseases as well! Type 1 diabetics generally aren't very sympathetic to type 2s; most of us with type 1 would cut off our left arms (or right arms, depending on which we favor) to make this go away. The two versions of diabetes are entirely different but, at the same time, very much alike.

Type 1.5 (aka the other diabetes)

Once there were only two types of diabetes; children mainly got one type and adults mainly got the other. Those lines are all blurred now and scientists have recently identified other diabetes subtypes beyond type 1 and 2. The most common of these is called latent autoimmune diabetes in adults (LADA), and it accounts for roughly 10 percent of people with diabetes, making it probably more widespread than type 1. It is a more slowly progressing variation of type 1 diabetes and is often misdiagnosed as type 2. Your immune system is attacking your pancreas but is still making insulin for a period of time. If you were eventually diagnosed with type 1 as an adult, but didn't need to take insulin the first 6 months or so, you might be a type 1.5. Good for you! You just got bumped up a half of a point!

Gestational Diabetes (aka the diabetes you will probably get rid of right after the baby is born)

For us to fully talk about diabetes, we must give a shout-out to a form of diabetes that you can get when you are pregnant. Medical experts don't exactly know what causes gestational diabetes either, but there are some clues. The same hormones from the placenta that help the baby develop can also block the action of the mother's insulin in her body. Thus, she develops insulin resistance, which makes it hard for the mother to use insulin. She may need up to three times as much insulin, but her body may not be able to produce it, resulting in gestational diabetes. Usually after a woman with gestational diabetes delivers her baby, the diabetes goes away. (I wish it worked that way with type 1.) Although, there *is* an increased risk for her to develop type 2 later on in life.

You are at the highest risk for gestational diabetes if you are older than twenty-five years when you get pregnant (um, that's most of us), have a family history of diabetes, gave birth in the past to a baby that weighed more than nine pounds, have high blood pressure, have too much amniotic fluid, were overweight before getting pregnant, or had a miscarriage in the past.

Gestational diabetes usually kicks in halfway through the pregnancy. All pregnant women should receive a glucose tolerance test between the twenty-fourth and twenty-eighth week of pregnancy to screen for the condition. Those who have risk factors for gestational diabetes may have this test earlier in the pregnancy. Women with type 1 diabetes get to skip that test. (Woo hoo—there ain't nothing new to find out in that department!) Don't worry, though; we make up for it with nuchal fold testings (high definition imaging which assesses chromosomal abnormalities as well as the quantity of fluid collecting at the base of the fetal neck), amniocenteses, and bimonthly doctor visits.

If you are diagnosed with gestational diabetes, good prenatal care is essential for a safe and healthy delivery.

Prediabetes

Although not an actual form of diabetes, you might have heard of *prediabetes*. That's when your fasting blood sugar numbers are on the high side but aren't high enough for you to be considered blessed with diabetes. People with prediabetes have impaired fasting glucose (100–125 mg/dL after an overnight fast) or impaired glucose tolerance (140–199 mg/dL after a two-hour glucose tolerance test). Some people have both. Approximately thirty-five million people ages forty to seventy-four have impaired fasting glucose, and sixteen million have impaired glucose tolerance. Because some people have both conditions, the total number of US adults ages forty to seventy-four with prediabetes comes to about 41 million. Unfortunately, a large number of prediabetics eventually become full blown diabetics.

Nearly twenty-nine million Americans have either type 1 or type 2 diabetes, which is a staggering 8.3 percent of the US population. It is estimated that 7 million people have diabetes and don't even know it and another 2 percent to 10 percent of pregnant women will develop gestational diabetes. That's way too many people when you add them all up. A new case of diabetes is diagnosed every thirty-seconds in the United States, and there are more than a staggering 350 million people in the world with diabetes—*three hundred fifty million.* Do you realize that that is more than the entire population of the United States? Can you imagine 350 million of *anything?* Unless you won one of the biggest lottery jackpots in history, my guess is that you cannot. When you feel all alone with your disease, take comfort in that

asking my sorority sisters at the table if anyone had ever experienced that sensation before without having taken any drug that might induce it. They all looked at me as though I were a tad unhinged, so I quietly ate my dinner, eventually felt better, and carried on.

That strange tingling in my mouth repeated itself often throughout the rest of my senior year. In addition, I experienced many other abnormal symptoms on and off, which earned me the title of "House Hypochondriac." One of these inexplicable ailments always seemed to occur during happy hour, and I would usually be the killjoy of the evening. A constant complainer and a killjoy—I must have been a real pleasure to be around! My friends and I usually spent our Friday evenings sipping margaritas and flirting with boys at one of URI's famous beachside happy hours. More often than not, I ended the party early with my insistence on leaving and getting food. I never knew what overcame me, but I knew I needed food that instant, or I would pass out with dramatic fanfare. Soon I started taking on the role of the designated driver every time we went out just so I could just take care of myself without being a pain in the ass. That worked out well for all of my friends to now have a personal chauffeur. I decided to diagnose myself with hypoglycemia because I thought it sounded cool at the time, *and* it seemed to make sense. No medical degree needed here—I knew it all! (For the record, I still do.)

As the resident house hypochondriac, I made many pilgrimages to the campus health services center. During every visit the doctor would recommend a checkup and a blood draw. I had been petrified of needles my entire life, and once I realized that I was an "adult" and *allowed* to turn down those dreaded finger pricks, I rejected blood work at my physical examinations every time. That was a foolish move on my part because I could have been diagnosed so much earlier, but instead, it took another two years. I showed them, didn't I?

While attaining my bachelor's degree, I somehow got pneumonia twice, once in my sophomore year and once in my junior year. Both times I went to the hospital directly from taking my LSATs (the test you take to apply to law schools). I never became a lawyer (thank goodness), but at one point I thought I wanted to, so I studied laboriously, spread myself too thin, didn't get enough sleep, had too much of a social life, and let my body wear down. This led to double pneumonia. I never fully recovered from it the first time, and it returned a few months later. My parents immediately yanked me out of school and made me come home for a few weeks to really rest and recover.

Why am I telling you this? Because I am convinced that that was what brought on this lovely disease that likes to wreak havoc with me every few days. I've always believed that the breakdown in my immune system triggered a cell that would not otherwise have been angered enough to turn on me. I am not sure why I even had the cell to begin with. I just got lucky, I guess. I also play Powerball religiously for that very reason. I am a lucky girl.

As a side note, if you are curious, my LSAT scores were stellar both times. I can't say the same for the people around me who wanted to ring my neck while I was coughing up a lung and disturbing them. I imagine by this time in their lives they are all doing whatever they wanted to do and have no hard feelings.

I went on to graduate *summa cum laude* from college with a degree in marketing, and I soon landed my first job—as a waitress at Bennigan's restaurant. Not exactly as impressive as I had planned, but sometimes you gotta do what you gotta do. I also thought that collecting pins with half-witted phrases on them to cover my mandatory suspenders was a fun thing to do. Many of them dealt with my love of chocolate, were snarky expressions to get customers to leave bigger tips, or a combination of both—"I accept tips in chocolate." I'm embarrassed to admit that one of my pins really said that.

That mindless gig lasted a few long and torturous months until I landed my dream job, which ended up not being so dreamy—but I'll save that for another book. I started on my career path doing public relations and marketing for a well-known fashion company. Before I started, I was required to have drug testing and get a physical examination. It was no surprise that I passed the drug test, but my blood panel results were another story. On the first day at my new job I received an alarming call from my doctor. He told me that my blood glucose level had come back at 424 and that I would be diabetic if it was truly accurate. He was shocked, as was I, because I didn't exhibit any common symptoms of the disease, and he really believed it could be a laboratory mistake. He ordered me to leave work immediately and get to the hospital for testing. This sounded serious, and I was beyond panic stricken.

Back to the laboratory I flew, caught up in a gaggle of nerves and shaking in my heart-patterned Prada shoes with the Chinese red lacquer heels. Back in the day I had a fabulous network of friends with "five finger discounts" in the fashion closets of luxury designers and I often benefited handsomely from it. Although much of D-day, also not-so-fondly known as diagnosis day, was a blur, I do remember exactly what I was wearing. It's kind of absurd that I can memorialize such a frivolous detail, but I always seem to associate major events with the clothing I wore.

Blood was again seized from my vein, and within twenty-four hours we had the results:

463! Yikes! Thank goodness WebMD wasn't around then, or I would have sent myself into an overresearched, overanalyzed tailspin. Instead, I was admitted to the hospital, hooked up to intravenous lines, given shots and icky food, and then officially given the devastating news: "Laura, you have diabetes." *Holy hell!*

Looking back, I was downing skim milk and pulp-free orange juice as though they were going out of style, but never did it cross my mind that I had diabetes. I just thought I was really thirsty! At the time of my diagnosis, my brother's longtime girlfriend and his very best friend both had type 1 diabetes, and I talked to them about it constantly. The Internet was only in its infantile stages, and social networking was still ten years away, so they were my only resource. I was very curious, always asking questions about taking shots and listening to their stories of passing out and almost passing out at various places. It was such a foreign concept to me. I really had no clue that, at the age of twenty-three, I could be diagnosed with type 1 diabetes, but here I was, slapped in the face with it. Time to stick the name tag to my chest: *Hello, my name is Laura, and I am a type 1 diabetic.*

I remember a few years before I was diagnosed, I was riding in an elevator, minding my own business and enjoying a Snickers bar. The doors opened a few floors before I had to get off, and an older gentleman walked in, took one look at me, and said, "If I ate that Snickers it would kill me." To which I replied, "Do you have a peanut allergy?" "No," he responded. "I'm diabetic." That memory raced through my head as I sat on the hospital bed after being diagnosed. Was this the end of sweet and tasty treats for me? Even worse, was I handed a death sentence if I couldn't resist a chocolate bar? Years later, I now feel bad for that man. He was completely uneducated about a condition he lived with every day, and for who knows how long. He had no idea that he could consume candy and still remain alive and kicking with the rest of us.

Right after I was diagnosed, I seemed to miraculously get better. I thought I had been cured; I honestly thought I was the first person on this planet to develop type 1 diabetes and then somehow get rid of it. I had always been a prodigy of sorts, so this made total sense to me. I even argued with my doctor that this could be possible. I *believed* I was cured. There's a first time for everything! What I really had experienced was called the "honeymoon phase," which is a span of time after diagnosis during which there is a huge decline in the need for insulin, and the diabetes almost goes away. Just like a honeymoon, that phase is temporary, and then real life kicks in. So much for my being able to shake the disease and become a case study and an anomaly of the medical and scientific world; the diabetes returned with a vengeance a few weeks later and has given me only one break since.

After I had my first baby, the same bewildering "cure" repeated itself. I didn't need insulin for four days after delivering. I was again convinced that I had been restored to my prediabetic self and somehow conquered the condition by having a baby. Stranger things have happened. My son once told me about a disorder called "alien hand syndrome," a neurological disease in which the afflicted person's hand appears to take on a mind of its own and can try to strangle the owner. If something like that actually exists, surely a random healing of diabetes must also be possible. This all makes sense to me in my head. Sometimes you want to believe something so much that you can actually talk yourself into it happening. It's like telling a lie enough times; after a while, you start to believe it too. Unfortunately, that wasn't the case. Having a baby does not cure diabetes. There would be a lot more babies in the world if it did!

Let's face it—I've got the sugar, and it's got me, and it's probably got you too. Let's try to make the best of it. Have fun with it, even. I've given my diabetic life theme songs: "Pour Some Sugar on Me" by Def Leppard for when I'm low, and "Sugarhigh" from the *Empire Records* soundtrack for when I am hyperglycemic. If you can't make yourself laugh, you are missing out on the best audience.

Chapter Three

You Know You're a Diabetic When...

di·a·be·tes (dī'ə
iabainein, to
used by an
chara ize
blood

I love labels, especially designer labels such as Gucci, Giorgio Armani, or Dolce & Gabbana. Truthfully, I don't even mind being labeled a bitch; I definitely have that in me. However, there is one label that I loathe: *diabetic*. I *hate* that diabetes has such a stigma attached to it. I do not want others to consider it a weakness. It bothers me when people say, "But you look healthy!" My response: "Well, of course I do, Sunshine. I work out, eat right, and take care of myself. I just happen to have a pancreas that decided to destroy itself, and now I have to take a jillion shots a day, count carbs, and see the doctor a few times a year." It's a completely manageable autoimmune disorder, but there's no denying that it takes considerable time, energy, and dedication to properly regulate it.

For the most part, this disease requires that you care for yourself, and it's the only disease that will never give you a break—*ever.* You can't put anything into your mouth, start exercising, drive a car, or go for a swim without checking your blood sugar or taking insulin. When you are diagnosed with diabetes, you have to make some big adjustments to the way you go about your life. Everything you do requires more thought, more preparation, and more action. Diabetes takes up a lot of time. It involves a lot of planning and it takes away a bit of life's spontaneity. It is now an integral part of what makes you, you. I have great respect for people living with any disease, especially those who will never know what it's like to live for a day without it.

When first given the "Scarlet D," most people go through five stages of dealing with diagnosis: *denial, information gathering, anger, sadness,* and then, finally, *moving on.*

> **Denial:** *This isn't happening to me. I feel fine, how can I possibly be sick?* You need to move past denial quickly, because blood tests are pretty accurate. I remember when I received the phone call letting me know my blood glucose results, my doctor and I

were both in the denial stage. He couldn't believe it either. If you want a second opinion, get another test. Then move on to the next stage of diagnosis.

Information Gathering: This is where search engines become your new best friend, and all of your human friends become experts on the subject as well. They offer you tons of advice and stories. Try not to listen too much to them, unless one of them happens to be diabetic.

Anger: Now you are pissed off. It's okay to get angry. Scream at your diabetes; tell it to go to hell. I still do that on occasion. Just don't let the anger take you over. It takes too much energy to be angry. You can put that energy to better use managing your diabetes. Remind yourself of the alternatives that come with not taking care of yourself. That should be enough to stop the rage from bubbling over.

Sadness: It's quite common to be blue after your diagnosis. *Why, oh why, did this happen to me?* You are grieving the loss of your old life. Try to not let it get the best of you, though. If you can't get out of your funk in a short time, please seek the help of a professional who can help you get past this stage. Diabetes almost doubles one's risk of depression.

Moving On: At some point, you should move into accepting the reality of your disease. It may take days, weeks, months, or years. You should start to feel well and be ready to face your diagnosis head on. That doesn't mean that you won't slip back into one of these stages every so often. You definitely will. Just keep your visit short. Rejuvenate by putting yourself into a peak state. Commit to a healthy lifestyle, think positively, and visualize your success in dealing with diabetes.

I experienced all of these stages in a relatively short window of time because it really only took about a month before I accepted the cards that I had been dealt. For the first few months, I treated it as something new and unique and took advantage of the attention it brought me. Then the novelty of it grew old fast. I've never let myself get depressed or drown in self-pity for too long. Once in a blue moon, I sometimes still get bitter and pissy and question why I got this disease. However, then I recover from my funk and consider myself lucky that it's fairly manageable, and that medicine has come a long way since the early twentieth century, or I'd be dead by now. My parents, on the other hand, felt extremely responsible for my diagnosis, and to this day, I think they still do. Technically, it *is* their fault (they gave me my DNA, after all), so I occasionally let them feel guilty just to keep things balanced and to assure me some added attention when I'm feeling particularly needy. Thanks, Mom and Dad—love you!

My parents really do hate to see me not feeling well and are especially concerned when I'm having a bad high or low. Oddly enough, I take warped pride in knowing that if any one of their five children had to get diabetes, they should be glad it was me because my four brothers have been notoriously irresponsible most of their lives. Studies have now found that although birth order alone is not a predictor of developing diabetes, being the first-born child in a family can contribute to a person's overall risk. As luck would have it, I was the first born. (Special note to my siblings: I know you are all on the right track now, so forgive me for bringing up the fact that I thought you were all delinquents and incapable of handling anything significant in your adolescent and young-adult years. Although, none of you are entirely compassionate to my high or low blood sugars even today, so I'd appreciate it if you worked on that. Many thanks.)

Over the years, I've had a few friends who unfortunately have developed different diseases. Many had to deal with god-awful treatments for their various issues, and I'm grateful that every one of them is okay and healthy now. They traveled a long and difficult road, but now they are able to put their sicknesses aside and carry on with their lives healthily and without ever having to think about what they went through every day. When raising money each year for diabetes research and awareness, I always try to tug on people's heartstrings with that very fact. Diabetes isn't going anywhere anytime soon. I don't remember my life before it, and I'm doubtful I will ever know what it's like to live without it. It's a daily struggle that never ends. It's overwhelming at times and definitely frustrating, and the only personal happiness I get from it is when I get a great A1C result (the test that shows your average blood sugar number over three months' time), and it feels as though I just aced a college exam. Hey, it's the little things.

So by now you have now admitted that you have diabetes. It's time to poke a little fun at yourself. Only a diabetic person will find the following list humorous, so don't try to entertain your friends.

You know you're a diabetic when:

1. You secretly like to see the reactions of strangers standing next to you when you say you are "high."

2. You ask for diet tonic and other sugar-free mixers at the bar or someone else's party.

3. You try on clothing in fitting rooms, not to see if the clothes fit but to see if you can hide your pump while wearing them.

4. You have the best candy drawer on the block or in the office, and people are constantly hitting up your stash—especially your children, if you have them.

5. Your refrigerator has a special section reserved just for insulin and you have at least one kitchen cabinet dedicated to diabetic supplies.

6. You buy handbags according to their ability to carry all of your medications, snacks, and devices.

7. You are an expert at dividing anything by fifteen, and you can count the carbs of just about anything you eat. It's as though you are a human Weight Watchers reference book.

8. People compare you to their diabetic cat.

9. You become slightly annoyed and oddly jealous at little kids gobbling up Halloween candy and birthday cake.

10. You have said some abominable swear words when your pump tubing has gotten caught on a doorknob—more than once.

Chapter Four

Stick It to Me

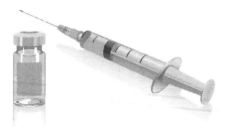

*G*reeks and Romans tested to see if they had diabetes by tasting their urine. Yum! If it was sweet and they were peeing just as quickly as they were drinking, almost like a siphon, they were able to diagnose themselves with the disease. In fact, they coined the name; *diabetes* is the Greek work for "siphon" or "to pass through," referring to the excessive urination associated with the disease and *mellitus* is the Latin term for "like honey," to reflect the sweet smell and taste of the patient's urine—hence, *diabetes mellitus.*

Since those ancient times, a multitude of medical devices have come on the market to help manage diabetes. There is no need to drink your own pee anymore, unless you are stranded in the desert somewhere and need hydration, but even then I don't recommend it. Then again, what do I know? Consult that crazy dude from *Man vs. Wild* if you have to make a decision like that.

Chances are, you are somewhat familiar with all the various diabetes technology out there. If not, you will be fully versed by the time you finish this chapter.

Glucose Meter

The glucose meter is a blood-sucking device that comes in all different shapes and sizes and reads the amount of sugar in your blood. You insert a test strip into the machine, prick your finger, squeeze a drop of blood onto the test strip, and wait for the meter to count down with your results. When you get your magic number, you can treat accordingly. This is a necessity if you are diabetic. If you are diabetic and don't own one, you are probably in more trouble than this book will ever be able to help with. Please get one. Have a spare one handy too. They decide not to work at the most inopportune times.

I have pricked myself more times than I could ever count. I'm not really sure I even have fingerprints anymore; the hundreds of thousands of needles that have darted unapologetically in and out of my poor fingertips seem to have destroyed them. This lack of identification would make me the perfect criminal, so that's something to fall back on if this book doesn't sell very well. It doesn't help that I am a rapid checker when my blood sugar numbers are out of whack; I need to know in what direction I'm headed. All that testing leads to my biggest diabetic pet peeve: the wasted test strip. This common diabetic occurrence happens quite frequently and can result from either accidentally applying blood before the meter is ready for it or testing without applying enough blood. If I am lacking in the red liquid, it is often the result of a dull needle or a chilly temperature. It drives me crazy to try to test my blood when my hands are cold; I just cannot get any blood out, no matter how hard I squeeze. Dead test strips can be found all over my home; I always tell people that if I am ever lost or go missing, they should look for the trail of test strips to find me. Sometimes, the polar opposite occurs, and I fear that I'll start leaking blood from holes that haven't closed up. There are times I prick my finger for a test, and hours later I can still squeeze the hole and gather enough blood to test again. (Bonus! No need to prick!)

I test my blood sometimes up to fifteen times a day. I'm not sure how you can get away with any less and still have tight control over this disease. I've tested my blood while driving my car, shopping, gambling, riding on a roller coaster, sitting in meetings, riding on a horse, standing on the top of the Empire State Building, and while rock climbing, on a ski lift, in a pool, the list goes on and on. My next book might be a photo essay of places my blood meter and I have traveled together. I spend so much quality time with it that I should give it a name. My seven-year-old suggests the name Vampire because it is always sucking my blood.

While a blood sugar monitor is certainly a life saver, it isn't always perfect. There is always a margin of error with meter readings and if you doubt the number at all, you should check again. I've had quite a few meter related stories over the years. Two in particular come to mind:

> I love to play tennis, and once I played an away singles match outside on a bitterly cold day. Because of the temperature, my glucose meter was not working, so I asked my opponent if we could play on an indoor court instead so that I could get a proper reading of my blood sugars. She refused and asked if I was a "type 3" diabetic. I told her there was no such thing, unless she was referring to the closest loved ones of a diabetic person, but she insisted that her son's girlfriend had type 3 diabetes, and that it was the worst form of diabetes to have. Her attitude and her ignorance threw me off my game, and she knew it; I ultimately lost the match. That was the first time my diabetes was used as a weapon against me.

> Besides being a tennis freak and a self-acclaimed dia-badass, I also love beauty products. I once used an expensive

moisturizer on my face, and when I tested my blood sugar a little while later, my reading was 425. I tested again and got close to the same reading, so I treated for it accordingly. What I didn't know was that one of the moisturizer's main ingredients was sugar, and I had some lotion residue on my fingers when I tested, causing the high reading. That is the closest that I have ever come to passing out; my blood sugar plummeted to nineteen and stayed below thirty for two hours, no matter what I did— scary stuff. When I came to my senses a few hours later, I realized that the only thing I had done differently was to use the moisturizer, so I put a bit on my finger and tested again: 375. Instead of making it my life's mission to get ingredients listed on the side of jars of facial cream, I decided to let it go and get in the habit of using alcohol swabs. This new habit lasted about a week.

Continuous Glucose Monitor (CGM)

A continuous glucose monitor, also called a CGM, reveals short-term trends in blood sugar as they happen. This relatively new device constantly measures glucose so you know your level at any given time. For people receiving intensive insulin therapy, seeing the dips or spikes that happen in response to food, medication, and exercise can help guide daily decisions. All CGMs are made up of three components: sensor, transmitter, and receiver. The sensor slips under the skin and is held in place by adhesive. A transmitter attaches to the sensor, relaying information to a handheld receiver or an insulin pump. CGMs measure the level of glucose in the fluid directly beneath the skin, which is similar to the blood glucose level a typical meter measures.

This is the biggest recent life changer in the world of diabetes technology. Continuous testing will truly change the face of this disease in the future, bringing us one step closer to the creation of an external, artificial pancreas that could someday automatically measure glucose and deliver insulin—much like the real thing. However, the first and second generation of CGMs got a bad rap because of accuracy and reliability issues. The newer ones are much more consumer-friendly and provide tremendously more information to aid users in managing their diabetes properly. I tried one of these babies for the short term just to get some trends with my blood sugar and found it to be very helpful. I am considering calling my insurance company to see if they cover long-term CGMs. You may want to give yours a call too.

Syringes and Insulin Vials

These represent the old-school diabetes treatment plan, but some people are stuck in their ways. The process may not be fancy, but it still gets the job done. The most ironic part of diabetes for me is that, until they became part of my regular life, I had always feared needles. I'd go as far as to describe it as a severe phobia. One of my earliest memories is of holding on for dear life to the leg of our living room's plastic-wrapped turquoise burnout velvet couch and not letting go until I was physically grabbed, smacked on the bum, and dragged to the doctor's office to get my immunizations. (Ah, the 1970s—a free-spirited time when you could hit your kids to make them succumb to your commands. Try that now and see how fast you are shunned by friends and neighbors and Child Protective Services arrives at your door.)

Incidentally, my fear of needles was replaced with a fear of flying, which I overcame as well, and is now replaced with a fear of spiders. I'm positive I will never get over this one; I will evacuate the premises for the life span of any big-enough spider I see crawling in my home.

Insulin Pump

First introduced over thirty years ago, the insulin pump is another all-in-one option that lets you go hands free, so to speak, and manage diabetes without injections (except for changing settings every few days). You inject insulin with the touch of a button. There are many pluses and minuses related to pump wearing: better blood glucose control is, of course, the biggest plus, and having an electronic device and tubing hanging from your side is the biggest minus. I wore one for eight years, so I've been on both sides of the fence. I have also had mine fall into the toilet on more than one occasion. Think about it—if it's attached to your hip or backside, you have to hold the thing in your hand while using the loo. Not an easy feat.

There are many different companies that manufacture pumps, and it's best to do a side-by-side comparison of features when choosing one. Factors such as screen size, infusion set choices, design, style, trend analysis, and overall pump size all are aspects to consider. Remember: you will have this pump for approximately five years, and if you choose the hot pink one, you might be sick of it very soon.

There is also a tubeless, lightweight pump option that you control the insulin infusion via a remote control. I also wore one of these when it first came out, but it was a little clunky for me when I tried it. They've recently made them much smaller, so I might be willing to give it another go!

The pump can change your life, helping you to live more freely. Among the many benefits are:

- Convenience with the times you choose to eat. Feel free to pop food into your mouth whenever the opportunity arises. Like a Boy Scout, you are always prepared.

- Quicker adjustments for changes in activity. You can cut it off on a moment's notice. There is never long acting insulin in your system, so once you suspend the pump, the insulin flow is cut off abruptly.

- Better insulin delivery and action and quicker response time to treat highs.

- Greater precision. That .1 unit feature really *does* come in handy.

- Easier problem solving. It does the math for you!

- Fewer morning highs. The constant basal keeps you level.

- Blood glucose swings are lessened. Balance is the key to life *and* to diabetes!

- Less hypoglycemia. Amen to that!

- Fewer supplies to lug around in your bag.

- You no longer have to lift your shirt or skirt up to take an injection (my personal favorite). I'm not a fan of flashing strangers.

To play devil's advocate, I have to let you know the cons of insulin pumps as well. There are, of course, a few negatives or else I'd still be wearing one:

- Scar tissue may build up around infusion sites, resulting in lumpy, bumpy skin.

- Air bubbles and clogs in the plastic tubing or infusion site can occur, resulting in an insulin deficit and an unnecessary high.

- Bleeding and hematomas at an infusion site can be uncomfortable and leave a nasty bruise.

- Your clothing choices have to be carefully thought out, as a pump is not as inconspicuous as one might first think.

- The tubing gets caught on things frequently.

- If you are very active, you might find that the pump can be awkward and clumsy during high-intensity workouts.

- You always have something hanging from you, and it frequently gets in the way.

Insulin Pen

My tool of choice is the insulin pen. I'm an all-in-one kind of woman, and the insulin comes already preloaded into this handy-dandy unit. There is no mixing or drawing medication into a syringe, and one pen lasts about a week. I figured out once that I have taken almost one hundred thousand insulin injections so far in my poor punctured body. That's more than the worst junkie and all of his junkie friends combined would ever dare to do. Where do I take all of these shots? I've always been partial to injecting in my stomach and the back of my hip because my legs and arms bruise up something fierce. I have no desire to look like the runner-up in the Ultimate Fighting Championship on top of feeling like a human pincushion.

I use an ultrafine needle with my pen, and it only hurts a little when I inject myself. I think I am desensitized to the feeling at this point. The insulin pen gives me freedom from being tethered to something all day and all night. I did love the pump with all of its benefits, including tighter control, but I have to say that I do not miss it. It's kind of like when your best friend comes to visit and you love having her around, there inevitably comes a time that you can't wait for her to leave and have your personal space and independence back again. That's my relationship with a pump.

Patch Pumps

This type of pump gets its own heading because, even though it's considered a pump, it is quite different from traditional pumps. Better known as a patch pump or tubeless pump, this revolutionary pump-like device has no tubing associated with it and is disposable. It is about the size of a credit card, but thicker. Patch pumps eliminate the need for some type 2 patients to take shots. The convenience, comfort, and discretion of infusing insulin can enhance quality of life for people with diabetes. Many type 2's skip insulin injections because of the pain or embarrassment of shots, so this is a good option. Other patch pumps are on the horizon as well, and we could very well see many more in the near future.

Emergency Glucose Kit

An emergency kit is an absolute necessity for any diabetic. At the first signs of hypoglycemia, an insulin user should treat it immediately by consuming carbohydrates to restore blood glucose to safe levels (thereby preventing progression to severe hypoglycemia). However, not all diabetics can feel and recognize the early signs, particularly when sleeping, and an emergency situation can develop in the blink of an eye. This can quickly lead to all those bad things I hesitate to mention. Stored in a conspicuous red package containing human glucagon, an emergency glucose kit does not require medical experience to use and can save your life. Get one. Tell your friends and family where it is and how to use it and then put it out of your mind because if you are prepared, you probably won't ever need it.

Ketone Test Strips

When your blood sugar runs high for an extended period of time, your body turns to reserves in order to get the energy it needs. The byproduct of this process is called ketones, and they can show up in your urine. Negative ketones are a good thing. Trace ketones means to treat your high blood sugar like you normally do, and moderate to large ketones means to treat and call your doctor ASAP. Your body could soon go into diabetic ketoacidosis (DKA). This is a serious and scary condition.

These strips are good to have around the house when your blood sugar escalates. The more tools you have on hand to monitor and manage your diabetes, the tighter your control will be.

Glucose Tablets

Although not really a tool, these tablets do come in handy a lot. I fought using them for many years, but when I finally realized that they are the fastest way to bring up your blood sugar in panic situations and are smaller than a juice box to carry around in your handbag, I gave in. The grape ones are the tastiest, and tropical fruit, although hard to find, are pretty palatable too.

Oral Medications

Healthy lifestyle choices, including diet, exercise and weight control, provide the foundation for managing type 2 diabetes. However, medications may be necessary to achieve target blood sugar levels. There are a variety of types available for a doc to prescribe, and frequently either one or a combination of a few help to manage levels very nicely. Sometimes a single medication is effective, and in other cases, a combination of oral medications works better. These miracle drugs can stimulate the pancreas to produce and release more insulin, inhibit the production and release of glucose from the liver, block the action of stomach enzymes that break down carbs, and improve the sensitivity of cells to insulin. There are even some non-insulin injectables that are being used that cause the body to release insulin or work with the insulin inside of the body to control blood sugar levels. Insulin is usually a last resort for a type 2.

Medical Alert Bracelets

We have come a long way since the stainless steel medic alert bracelets of yesteryear. I love the retro vibe they give off, but there are plenty of other jewelry options to choose from to fit your distinct style. It's a wise choice to wear one on the chance occasion that you are alone and have some sort of diabetic event. You wouldn't want a bystander to assume you are intoxicated or on some sort of acid trip. If bracelets are not your thing, maybe tattoos are? I've been toying with the idea of getting one inked on the inside of my right wrist. It's a badge of honor as far as I'm concerned. Although, my fear is that I would then feel like I'd also have to get my kids names inscribed somewhere on my body and I would slowly morph into a human Etch A Sketch.

Chapter Five

A Love/Hate Relationship

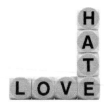

Something guys might not relate to when it comes time to lugging all those diabetic supplies and equipment around is that you can no longer use a tiny purse when you are all dressed up. I love those precious dainty bags that can only fit a lip gloss, a key, and a credit card, but there's definitely no room for all my monitoring swag. Instead I carry a big feed-sack around, filling it with all my diabetic paraphernalia and anything else I can possibly stuff in it, including tennis balls, my iPad, all sorts of receipts, and *six* different lip glosses (six lip glosses *might* be a little excessive, but I never know what kind of mood I'm going to be in!). If I have the room in my bag, trust me: I'll be hoarding lip glosses.

The "Hate" List

The size of our bags isn't the only daily frustration that we diabetics experience. Oh no, the list is endless. Here is my list of "hates":

- I hate when I take a shot, and the insulin balls up under my skin like a hard little marble is in there. I then have to spend hours wondering if I'll really get the intended full dose of insulin and how long it will take to soak into my bloodstream.

- I hate when I pull out the needle and have a bleeder and what is sure to be a nasty little bruise afterward. Even worse is when the hole shoots out blood as though I just hit an artery. I always seem to have a white shirt on when that happens.

- I hate when I remove an infusion set, and the blood pours out as though I've been bitten by a vamp from *True Blood*. Those gushers can be very dramatic when they start squirting like the geyser in Yellowstone National Park.

- I hate when I forget to change the needle in my poker (or I was too lazy to do so). It hurts like hell when I stab myself with a dull point, yet I'll do this at least ten more times until I finally change out the lancet.

- I hate when people joke about diabetes. Someone who didn't know I had the disorder once tried to be witty while I was eating a cupcake: "That looks like diabetes in a wrapper." I told him to take a closer look at what I was wearing, because that's what diabetes in a wrapper looks like.

- I hate that diabetes makes you wait. You are always on its schedule.

- I hate when I am giving myself a shot in the middle of the night while half asleep and I don't take the cap off of the needle but I assume I've taken my shot anyway. What an unpleasant surprise that is to wake up to in the morning!

- I hate when I rage bolus, taking repeated doses of insulin because my blood glucose won't come down, yet knowing full well that I'll end up with a low later.

- I hate when I have a high, and my eyes become blurry, and I feel as though I've just had an emotional cry.

- I hate it when I get the tubing of my insulin pump lassoed on a cabinet knob as I walk past, especially when it results in the entire setting getting ripped from my stomach. My endearing term for that is "pump lassoing." I'm currently on a pump holiday, and that is one of the reasons why. After eight years of pump wearing I also got tired of having something hanging from my stomach twenty-four hours a day, seven days a week. Although I am a big fan of the pump and how much better control you can have on it, I am also a fan of fitted shirts and dresses, both of which are a fashion disaster when you are hooked up to that thing. You also cannot turn over easily in the middle of the night when you are sleeping, and going swimming at the beach or a public pool always leaves you open for stares about the large bandage on your midsection. That said, I'm considering going back on the pump in the very near future. You have to keep mixing it up.

- I hate when I forget to take my long-acting shot at night because I have taken so many shots throughout the course of the day, and they all seem to swirl together in a foggy haze. I also hate when I double down and take shots twice for the same exact reason. Please remember, I cannot blame this forgetfulness on too many lows; my mental functioning has remained untouched, according to scientific study.

- I hate when I dry spike and stab myself repeatedly and cannot get enough blood out of my finger to get an accurate reading.

- I hate when someone complains about getting a flu shot at the doctor once a year.

- I hate the blood I find on my sheets from middle-of-the-night testing.

- I hate when nondiabetic people try to educate me on the disease. An associate did that to me recently, as though I had no clue about something I have lived with for almost two hundred thousand hours. Yeah, it's all new to me. Please educate me with all of your wisdom.

- I hate stepping on a needle cap in the dark. It feels just like stepping on a Lego, and that hurts wicked bad.

- I hate when I order unsweetened tea, and the waitress brings me the sugar loaded version. Not everyone in the South drinks sweet tea, you know! When I dramatically exclaim that she's trying to kill me it's kind of fun.

- I hate that I have to always second-guess every high I have, wondering if the meter reading was accurate and if the insulin really went in or not. Do I need to take a follow-up shot?

- I hate packing for a week's vacation but taking a month's worth of supplies.

- I hate being asked to put my phone away when it's really my pump, and I have to explain that.

- I hate getting my luggage searched at airports because of needles or juice boxes.

- I hate the little circular black and blues I have all over my hips and stomach.

- I hate injecting in public and having someone tell me that needles really make them uncomfortable. In my head, I am making a mental note not to be as discreet about the next one.

- I hate getting a bad low at the worst possible moment. That's the story of my life. Even worse, I hate sounding like a babbling idiot when I have that bad low.

- I hate being woken up by a low blood sugar. Although that certainly beats the dangerous alternative: being visited by the Sugar Reaper.

- I also hate having to wake up during the night to check my sugar to begin with. I have not had a full night's sleep in twenty years, and I sleep so lightly now that I never really feel refreshed in the morning.

- I hate that I have no recollection of my life without diabetes. I kind of equate it to not remembering what life was like before my children were born. The difference is, however, I like my children. Diabetes, not so much.

My complaining has come to an end, even though I know you are probably sitting there nodding your head along in agreement with every word I've said. Let's move on to what I love about diabetes:

The "Love" List

- I love when my glucose reading is 111. I always make a wish. For a cure.

- I love educating and helping others.

- I love being a role model for other people with diabetes.

- I love receiving a stellar A1C result.

- I love having an excuse to buy candy. Especially holiday-themed sweets. I love chocolate at Valentine's Day, candy corn around Halloween, and Peeps and jellybeans at Easter time. Mixing it up keeps me from being bored and keeps my mouth entertained.

- I love the confidence, determination, and perseverance that this disease has brought me.

The list isn't very long. There's not too much to love, but the truth is that although diabetes doesn't define me, it has sculpted me into the person that I am today. It's made me tough, both mentally and physically. It has given me credence in knowing that I have control over my body and how it looks and feels. It's taught me discipline and acts as a symbol not for someone who is sick but rather for someone who is healthy and not easily knocked down. It has also made me realize that there is no such thing as failure, and every second of every day is another opportunity to begin again.

Chapter Six

Busting Diabetic Myths

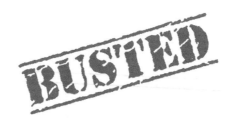

*m*yths are never completely accurate but always seem to have a small element of truth to them, so people believe them. I never fell into that trap, and I do not want you to either.

Here are the top 10 things nondiabetic people should know about us sugary sweet ones:

1. Yes, it hurts. It's a needle going into my flesh. What do you think it feels like?

They say a stupid question deserves a stupid answer, or is it that there is no such thing as a stupid question? Either way, asking if a needle hurts when you plunge it into your skin is like asking me if I want a martini. Duh.

2. No, my diabetes won't go away. You also cannot cure it with vitamins or supplements.

By the time someone is diagnosed with diabetes, that person has lost a major portion of his or her beta cell function. Unless you have developed a method of regrowing those beta cells, fixing the broken protein-folding sequences, and/or re-regulating the hormones that interrupt insulin-secretion and reception, you have not cured any form of diabetes. To cure type 1 diabetes, not only would you have to regrow the lost beta cells and make sure they're producing insulin correctly, but you would also have to stop and reverse the autoimmune response that causes diabetes to happen in the first place. Of course, fixing that autoimmune response may potentially be the key to "curing" a number of other autoimmune conditions too—bonus! Autoimmune conditions like type 1 diabetes can be triggered at any age, and once triggered, they don't *un*trigger. Children with type 1 diabetes do not "outgrow" diabetes in the manner that children may "outgrow" certain types of asthma and allergies. However, all of that said, type 2's do have a shot at making diabetes go away through diet and exercise.

3. No, I do not need candy to fix my high blood sugar or insulin to fix my low.

I do not have a soft spot in my heart for people who know nothing about diabetes and have the nerve to criticize me about the way in which I take care of myself. Back when I was working as the marketing director for a huge lingerie company in New York, I had a severely low blood sugar while I was at an event with the chief executive officer of the company. She was a relatively famous woman, a D-list celebrity of sorts, who shall remain nameless. Her reaction to my condition was, "Take some insulin, Laura. You should really take better care of yourself." *Good idea, oh ignorant one, I'll take more insulin and put myself into a hypoglycemic coma.* Geez. Even though I was half out of it with my low, I still had it in me to want to pop her in the face. Lows do get you a little cranky and somewhat aggressive, it seems.

4. No, eating too much sugar does not cause diabetes, and eating properly doesn't necessarily make it easier to manage.

So many factors affect blood sugar readings. Among them is not only what you are eating, of course, but also what exercise you do, how often you do it, any other medications you might be taking, what stress you are under, if you are physically sick, and, if you are a woman, what day of your menstrual cycle you are on. When my blood sugar is completely normal and reacts perfectly to how many carbs I just consumed, I am sometimes taken completely off guard. 329? Where did *that* come from? Do what you can do and give it your all, and don't sweat the occasional bad (or awful) reading. Just take care of it and move on.

5. No, you can't catch it.

Diabetes is a disorder and cannot be passed on like the common cold. Diabetes is not communicable: you cannot "catch" diabetes from anyone (not even if you come into direct contact with that person's blood). Diabetes is a syndrome that describes the body's inability to properly process glucose and regulate serum glucose levels. It is a direct response from your body to conditions within your body.

6. No, you do not have to be fat to have diabetes.

Diabetes does not discriminate. Just because your aunt has diabetes and weighs three hundred pounds does not mean that every diabetic person is overweight. People have really gone as far as to say to me, "I thought diabetics were all fat."

Although overeating *can* cause you to gain weight and fat cells *can* secrete hormone-like substances that interfere with normal glucose regulation, your *diet* is not the cause of your diabetes (but it *can* make your diabetes worse). Many people who are overweight or obese do not have, and never will develop, diabetes. People of normal weight who have never been overweight in their lives can develop type 2 diabetes. In fact, most type 1 diabetics are of normal weight or even a bit on the thin side.

7. Yes, I am diabetic and yes, I can eat that.

Remember that guy in the elevator who thought he could never eat a candy bar again? Well, he was wrong, and it is such a shame that he is in the dark about that. Of course you can enjoy a bolus-worthy sweet treat. You just need to make sure you cover it with enough insulin, a bit before the indulgence, so you don't have that quick spike up that you otherwise would normally follow with a big fat shot of insulin and then be sucker-punched with a bad low. It's a vicious, repetitive cycle.

Truthfully, doctors should be blamed for that man's lack of knowledge. So many doctors tell their patients that they must stay away from sugar in *any* form, including foods that will eventually turn to sugar, such as spaghetti with marinara sauce or savory garlic bread. Those carbohydrate-filled foods raise blood sugar as much as a fudge brownie. The truth is, however, if you take insulin you can eat almost anything you want (in moderation) as long as you pay close attention to carbohydrate counting.

8. Yes, I can get health insurance.

It has been proven that people with diabetes take better care of themselves than the general population, which brings me to the next false statement, *that a diabetic person can't get health insurance.* Although it is a preexisting condition, and insulin and test strips cost an arm and a leg, you can still obtain health insurance - especially now with the Affordable Care Act. Don't give it a second thought when you are switching jobs or have to go out and buy your own because of unforeseen circumstances. Keep in mind that, although you can get health insurance, this does not eliminate the possibility that you might run out of test strips one month and your insurance company will not let you get a refill of your prescription because it's too early. Those frustrating insurance trials and tribulations happen often enough and usually result in unnecessary pulling of one's own hair and hyperventilating.

9. No, I don't want to hear about your "friend of a friend" who had diabetes and died.

We have all have heard the horror stories before. Someone you barely know, when they find out you are diabetic, feels the need to inform you about their "friend" who died from diabetes. They tell you half of a story, and when you ask them specific questions about this friend, they can't answer them. You rarely die from the disorder itself, but you can become seriously ill or die from complications that arise by not taking care of yourself. That's why I prefer to call this disease "live-abetes." I'm living with it, not dying from it.

10. No, my children don't have it, and I wish you wouldn't ask, especially when there is no wood around for me to knock on.

Remember how I mentioned that no one in my family had diabetes? Everyone thinks that the disease is inherited. The questions "Who else in your family has diabetes?" and "Do your children have diabetes?" get tiring and upsetting when I hear them from anyone who finds out that I have it. Those are the first two questions people ask. Many of you reading this book likely already have diabetes, so you know better. Alert all of your friends and family; go ahead and put it as your Facebook status, Twitter update or Instagram photo message to educate others. "Newsflash: You can have type 1 diabetes and not have inherited it from anyone in your family, and it's not a guarantee that your kids are going to get it either." Maybe that will go viral and stop the recurring, painful questions.

Chapter Seven

How Low Can You Go?

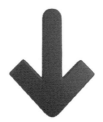

*H*ypoglycemia can be fierce and unrelenting. You can't process information normally. You have to stop what you are doing, devour something carb filled, and wait for it to get better. Many times you gluttonously overeat because of the hunger and confusion it riddles you with, and minutes later you roller-coaster back with a bad high. When your sugar level tanks, you often spend precious time lollygagging in the candy aisle, unable to decide what to buy or even remember your name. Lows are a beastly byproduct of living with diabetes.

Many times a blood sugar dip also inconveniences those around you. If you are really lucky, however, you will have a significant other who is more than happy to help get you out of the depths of a low; these wonderful people are often referred to as "type 3 diabetics" because they have to deal with the idiosyncrasies of their diabetes partner. My type 3 diabetic sweetheart loads up my nightstand with sweet snacks, juice, and glucose tablets every evening. These "treats" come in very handy at four in the morning, when running downstairs to the refrigerator is the last thing you want to do (and the last thing your type 3 wants to do as well).

When that scenario does occur, you tend to eat more than you should. It's best to ration out your bedside snacks in groups of fifteen carbohydrates each. It's much easier not to have to think about how many carbs you are consuming when your brain feels like it is covered in a heavy layer of moss.

When you get a really crazy low, you feel crappy for a little while after. Maybe you will have a headache or will be slightly confused or not feel like yourself. To be honest, I have lows a lot; probably more than the average bear. Unfortunately, there's a rumor out there that hypoglycemia kills brain cells. Even though it might feel that way temporarily, it's really not the case. Tests have proven that repeated bouts of hypoglycemia will not permanently damage an adult brain and do not cause bad complications (however the older you get, the more careful you have to be with lows). It's another story with children, because their brains are still developing, but adults will have no loss of mental functioning. So don't throw out that excuse when you forget to meet your friend after work, or you can't help your nephew with his third grade math homework. The truth is that a severe low can make you feel helpless and frustrated. I can cite so many instances of those very feelings. The two that stick out in my head are what I less-than-fondly refer to as "the Godiva incident" and "the master disaster."

The Godiva Incident

It was Christmas time in New York City, the most wonderful time of the year. I was window shopping on Madison Avenue when my glucose levels took a nasty turn for the teens. I had nothing in my handbag to combat the crash. Everywhere I turned I saw nothing but high-end designer retail boutiques. Normally, that would be my description of heaven, but at that moment I started to panic. There wasn't even a pretzel stand nearby where I could grab a quick soda. Anyone who knows me would recognize that I had to be in complete survival mode to even consider drinking a Coke, Pepsi, or even a Sprite. I've never had a sip of those syrupy, sweet, carbonated drinks in my entire life. I know that sounds a bit crazy, but just lump it into the fact that I also hoard lip gloss and shoes. It's not completely normal, but then again, I've never claimed to be.

As I was sweating profusely and running in slow motion on the crowded sidewalk, desperately looking for something to eat or drink to raise my blood glucose, I spotted a Godiva Chocolate boutique. I propelled myself through the door and pushed ahead of everyone on line. Keep in mind, it was the holiday season, and there was an absurdly long line of people buying candy as gifts for people for whom they either didn't know too well or didn't care to think of a creative gift. I pleaded with the guy behind the counter. "Give me anything. Just give me something. Chocolate. Anything. Please. Now." He stared at me as though I had two rhinestone rainbow horns sticking out of the top of my head, but I think he quickly caught on that this was some sort of emergency. Either that or I was robbing the place. Regardless, he quickly started handing over truffles, caramels, and chocolate-dipped pretzels, and I think I swallowed them all whole.

As a diabetic you know (or will quickly find out) that chocolate isn't the ideal food for bringing your sugar up rapidly because it is also filled with fat. However, desperate times called for desperate measures in this case. It took a while for my levels to get back to normal, but when I was finally able to put together a sentence, I thanked the lifesaver who fueled me with chocolate and gave him a pithy explanation for my erratic behavior. That also seemed to pacify all the testy people on line that I offended when I deliberately cut ahead of them. Where was their Christmas spirit? By the way, my blood sugar registered as an eighteen that day. That was the lowest I have ever seen it plummet.

That very same scenario (sans a Godiva boutique) has repeated itself many times in my life. None has been quite as melodramatic as that particular occasion—until the master disaster.

The Master Disaster

My first-ever public speaking event was an informational lecture to a master's program at Columbia University on the topic of public relations. I am normally not a very nervous speaker, so it struck me as strange that I felt so jittery that day before going on stage. I had checked my blood glucose before going out, and the meter said 120. Perfect. Maybe it was a bit of stage fright?

I was formally introduced, strolled on stage, and started my dog-and-pony show. I think I said the first few sentences clearly and distinctly, but then I lost my train of thought and immediately turned into a colossal, garbled, hot mess. Before I knew what was happening, the words "I'll be right back" came flying from my mouth as I hightailed it off of the stage. It was my worst nightmare come true. In a flash I checked my blood sugar, and my very bizarre behavior was explained—a lovely low of thirty-five. There was no time for humiliation to set in; I had to act swiftly.

I bolted to my handbag, consumed as many SweeTarts as I could, and waited until I stopped seeing spots and started seeing levels above ninety. Amid some whispering from the crowd, I ultimately made my way back out on stage again. Instead of keeping my tail between my legs, I committed to address this head on. I told the crowd I was diabetic and was under the attack of some overeager insulin. I cracked some more jokes at my expense and carried on. What choice did I have?

That isolated event built up my confidence and gave me so much of the character I have today. I recommend you all try it; it's the diabetic person's equivalent of being naked in front of a crowd.

Sometimes with diabetes, though, we take two steps forward and one step back in our outlook on the disease. Very recently I was invited as the guest of a prominent celebrity psychiatrist to a benefit for Alzheimer's Association. He spoke about the connection between type 2 diabetes and high blood sugar numbers and the onset of

Alzheimer's. I stood and asked, "If I am a type 1 diabetic, and I maintain very tight control to make sure to stay away from highs, how are the inevitable lows affecting me?" His answer was an obnoxious, "Horribly!" This guy happened to be about five-one with what I am sure was a Napoleon complex as I stood next to him, all six foot of me in some killer boots (I told you I remember what shoes I am wearing at all times). I think he just wanted to make me feel bad and the best he could do was to take a jab at my condition. As type 1 diabetics, highs and lows are part of our daily existence. I've since decided to cross experimental psychiatrists off of my list of people I want anything to do with.

The Lowdown on the Lows

What's truly interesting about low blood sugar is that the symptoms are never the same from person to person or episode to episode. There are many types of lows, and you can experience a different one every day or even a few simultaneously. Which types of lows can you relate to?

The Underwater Dream World Low: Your brain is all fuzzy, and you feel as though you are moving in slow motion. It is absolutely impossible to focus on anything.

▼ *The Surprise Low:* You've randomly tested your blood, and to your bewilderment, it is below fifty-five. You don't have any signs or symptoms that you are entering dangerous territory.

▼ *The Sweaty Low:* Clammy, hot, and uncomfortable are the best words to describe your body. It's made even worse when the temperature outside is above seventy degrees and you are doing *anything* except sitting motionless in front of a fan.

▼ *The Tingly-Lipped Freaky Low:* It feels as though your lips, tongue, and sometimes even your chin can vibrate off of your face. It is the most peculiar sensation, and one that could never be replicated even if you tried.

▼ *The Cranky Low:* Premenstrual syndrome (PMS) has got nothing on the cranky low. You snap at everyone and anyone in your vicinity. You also may swear, scream, and overall have rage-like behavior.

▼ *The Hypo Hangover Low:* Diana Ross may have had the sweetest hangover that she didn't want to get over, but a hangover from a bad low feels almost like one from alcohol—except you weren't enjoying yourself the night before.

▼ *The Double-Dipper Low:* You finally come out of your low and think that things are stable when another one slams you right back down. Now you have to ride out this wave too. This situation is not limited to only two instances; the fun can continue for hours depending on how generous you were with your insulin earlier.

↓ *The Nocturnal Low*: You shoot up, wide awake, in the middle of the night and know without even testing that you are hitting rock bottom. The Sugar Reaper has come to attack. Time to chug some juice!

↓ *The Full But Still Have to Eat Low*: What a drag! You just ate a big meal and your belly is full, but you overbolused, and now you have to eat *more* to fend off the low.

↓ *The Unconscious Low:* This one is self-explanatory and the very worst of all the lows. Next...

↓ *The Numb Body Low:* This usually happens after you have been low for quite some time, for instance, when you are sleeping and do not realize it. You awaken with a startle and, without even testing, quickly consume juice or whatever happens to be next to you. As you wait for glucose to go back into your cells, every extremity—including but not limited to your legs, arms, face, and ears—feels as though it is being stabbed with little pins and needles.

⬇ *The Meet Your Liver Low*: Next to the Unconscious Low, this is my least favorite one. Your liver has announced to your internal organs that you aren't supplementing your body with sugar fast enough, and it decides to intervene by spilling out stored glucose into your bloodstream. Your body will always respond with a skyrocketing high reading sometime soon after. The one-sided conversation I have with my liver usually goes something like this: "Mind your own business liver, I will be fine on my own. I might have a new admiration for your functions if you prevent me from passing out, but I'd appreciate you keeping to the activities you were intended to do. Continue cleaning out toxins from my blood, and I'll take care of the diabetes side of things."

⬇ *The Race to the Finish Line Low*: Have you ever tried to beat out a low? You know you have one looming, but you want to finish up whatever task you are working on before you go tend to it. What I have come to realize is that this is a very senseless thing to do. You get nothing accomplished. I'm working on this point myself (sort of) right now. My blood sugar is sixty, but I want to finish this chapter.

Lows come in all shapes and sizes, and most likely, you have experienced your own unique low as well. See if you can come up with a name for your next one and try not to use profanities.

Chapter Eight

I've Got High Hopes! Yeah, High Hopes!

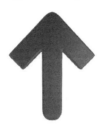

*W*hat goes down, must have started up. The only thing I hope for when my blood sugar is high is for it to decline, *pronto!*

Our pancreases are broken. Because of this, we have blood sugars that are less than perfect. Many times our readings are much too high. The technical name for this is *hyperglycemia.* Sometimes the amount of glucose in your blood can even skyrocket to dangerous levels. The sad fact is that every person with diabetes has experienced highs more times than he or she would probably care to admit. Highs are frustrating and time consuming—they slow you down, depress you, and can make you feel defeated. Plus they are dangerous and can do all sorts of torturous things to your body.

When you first realize you have a high blood sugar, you know that it's not going to be an easy fix. Highs can take hours to come down. If you eat or drink anything it will just drag out the process longer. This is one of the most frustrating things about being a diabetic. I like an instant solution, and that's why lows are so much more appealing to me. I'll take a 58 over a 258 any day of the week. Highs result in psychotic repeated glucose testing to see if the numbers are starting a downward trend. It is impossible to put your high sugar level out of your mind; it's a recurring thought that will not take a back seat to any other thought in your head.

Everything slows down when you get a high. Reflexes are sluggish, your mind is drowsy, and you feel that overall you are in a sugar-induced fog. Many times all you want to do is nap, but you can't. Unfortunately, life does not come to a halt just because your blood sugar is high. Instead, life goes on at an accelerated pace, and you have to just keep up. The perfect example of not being able to hit the pause button was when I was competing in the United States Tennis Association (USTA) City Finals. (I realize I have more than a few tennis stories, and I apologize if you don't share my obsession with it, but tennis is symbolic for so many other life experiences. I mean, how many times in your life you have said, "The ball is in your court?")

I was playing singles, and it was about ninety-five degrees. That morning I had eaten something that didn't agree with the amount of insulin I had shot up (go figure). I started off playing with a high of two hundred, which was not a big deal because I feel my best when my blood sugar is about 160 and I am exerting tremendous amounts of energy. Between the first and second set my level creeped up to just under three hundred. I gave myself a hefty shot in the tush and continued my play. Soon into that set I started to feel very woozy, and I thought for sure it was the heat because I was sweating like I was on a safari in Africa with no shade over my jeep.

I checked my glucose again between the second and third sets, and it was 423. The adrenaline in my body, combined with my poor breakfast choice, must have been the cause of this unusual high. This was not good at all. I was playing in a championship game and it was up to me to bring my team to the state finals. Contrary to any advice my doctor would have given, I continued to play—regardless of the fact that I couldn't breathe well, I felt terrible, and all I could do was think about my skyrocketing blood glucose. I wasn't going to let diabetes make this decision for me. I lost in a tiebreaker in the third set. I do not like losing; I am always out there to win, and now I had nothing to show for pushing myself beyond my physical limitations. Would I do it again? Probably. I know my endocrinologist is reading this book, so I am going to add in (for legal and medical reasons) to never, ever do this to yourself. It is not healthy. Do not exercise if your blood sugar is sky high, and especially not if you are spilling ketones.

What is the lesson learned here? For one, obviously I do not always make the best decisions. Continuing to play wasn't very smart. Yet there was more to this than just winning the match: I did not want to let diabetes get the best of me. None of us should. Don't let it be a crutch or an excuse. Keep forging ahead and keep your determination focused and your attitude positive. It's not always easy. This disease is a part of everything that makes you *you*, but don't let it dominate your life.

There is one tiny device that does try to exert some control over us, though: the blood glucose meter. I have a love/hate relationship with that little meter. On particularly bad days it's a judge of my self-worth. I feel like a terrible person when the results are high. I almost can hear my meter preaching, "Another high blood sugar? What did you eat this time?" and "What do you expect when you eat a cupcake, idiot?" Throughout high school and college, I never came close to failing a test. Yet I repeatedly fail my glucose test a few times a week. How frustrating! Not only that, but every time I have a bad number, I am reminded that yes, I have diabetes. I am more than a number though. It is not a measure of my self-worth or my overall management. It's just a blip on the radar.

In the same vein, when I have a particularly unusual day brimming with all perfect numbers, I think I am cured. I envision myself being the first person in the world who has been miraculously cured of diabetes without an islet cell transplant. As farfetched as it sounds, I still have just a wee bit of faith that my fairy tale might come true. That's right. Some women dream of knights galloping in on white horses to whisk them away to become a princess. I dream of life without diabetes. Seems fair.

We all know that high blood sugars cause damage to our bodies over time. Our eyes, kidneys, circulatory system, heart, you name it, it's all affected by poor care of your diabetes. The truth is that all of those pesky high blood sugar numbers are just little pieces of a big puzzle. They are just numbers. As long as you get them down quickly, you are doing all you can to stay as healthy as you can. Check your blood frequently and address issues as they arise. We all have so many numbers that are normal too, so don't get discouraged when you have a bad day or week.

Up, Up, and Away

Just as there are many types of lows, there are endless breeds of highs as well. So many external factors can adversely affect your efforts to control your blood sugar levels including stress, hormonal changes, periods of growth, physical activity, medications, illness, and fatigue. It's truly amazing when you get a normal reading! See how many of these highs you have experienced:

↑ *The Didn't Shoot Up Enough High*: This one is completely your fault. You ate too much and didn't take the right amount of medicine to cover it. It often happens when you dine out at a restaurant or go to a party. You never know what ingredients have been used and how much of them were in what you ate. This is also fondly known as *The Crap Shoot High*.

↑ *The Ate Too Many Carbs High:* This is kind of your fault again. You overindulged—ate too much pasta, too much bread, or too many sweets. It happens to the best of us! Don't beat yourself up.

↑ *The Too Much Adrenaline High:* The adrenaline hormone is great in the sense that it helps to increase courage and overcome fears, but it also raises blood sugar in the blink of an eye. If you have ever played a physically competitive sport, had a huge presentation at work, ridden a really scary roller coaster, or gotten into a car accident, then you know all about the Too Much Adrenaline High. Any activity that produces excitement, fear or danger can escalate your blood sugar, and quickly!

↑ *The Stress-Induced High*: If you have ever been super angry, the kind of angry that is accompanied by steam coming out of your ears, or if you have just had one of those days in which *everything* is driving you nuts (who hasn't?), then you have experienced the Stress-Induced High. In comparison with the other highs, this one is the most exasperating, because your high resulted from being pissed off, not from eating something decadent. When my blood sugar is low, my children want to know if they should get me angry so it goes back up again. It's a valid thought, but I have yet to allow them that indulgence.

↑ *The Sick as a Dog with the Flu High*: You can't eat, you are throwing up, and you are practically begging someone to put you out of your misery. The cherry on top is that your blood glucose is out of control. You might even have ketones in your pee, in which case call your doctor immediately. The only thing that could possibly make it worse is all of those bolus corrections you are taking end up resulting in a low, and you now have to *eat* something to bring it back up. Then you throw up again, and the cycle continues. I shudder just thinking about it.

↑ *The No Good Reason High*: No explanation. No excuse. No motive. No logic behind it. It just makes no sense whatsoever. This is also known as the *Twilight Zone High* (cue the theme song).

⬆ *The Premenstrual High:* Think of it as diabetic PMS. You still get bloated, acne, fatigue, food cravings, mood swings, and irritability, but that's not all! You are also the recipient of sky-high blood sugar readings as well. It never fails; three days before you start your period your numbers start creeping up. Catapulting to the three- or four-hundred range is not unheard of and makes you even crankier. It's best to avoid loved ones for seventy-two hours.

⬆ *The Good Morning High*: You wake up to check your blood at 4 am and score a sublime 105, only to get out of bed at 7 am with a 245. That's called the *dawn phenomenon*. It sounds poetic, but it's just completely frustrating.

⬆ *The Dry Eye High*: Your blood sugar is high and you know it, because as you blink, your lids feel like they have sugary sandpaper on the inside. You feel as though you need some eye drops, but when you use them they don't really help. This feeling goes away immediately upon your sugar returning to normal.

⬆ *The I Just Want to Take a Nap High*: You are soooooo sleepy. You have no energy, and all you want to do is lie on the couch or crawl into bed and snooze off the high.

⬆ *The Stripper High*: Clothing is peeled off as your sugar climbs higher. How did it get so damn hot in here?

↑ *The Shot in the Dark High*: You woke in middle of the night to check your blood, found it to be high, and groggily corrected for it in the darkness of the room. Only problem is, after the shot, you cannot say for sure if you took the cap off of your needle or not. You wake up two hours later with an even higher number.

We have all experienced the highest of highs and the lowest of lows. To really appreciate those normal readings, you have to have been at both ends of the spectrum. Consider your outrageous highs and senseless lows as recurring rites of passage. After all, if you didn't have them, you wouldn't be diabetic!

Over the duration of writing this book, which took two years, my blood sugar was above two hundred one hundred ten times and dropped below fifty eighty-five times. I kept track.

Chapter Nine

Do you Speak Carbonese?

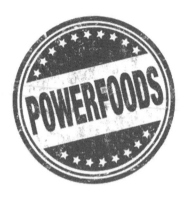

*B*efore the discovery of insulin in 1921 (thank you, Frederick G. Banting & Charles H. Best), doctors used to put their patients on starvation (or near-starvation) diets, recommending they only eat foods such as oatmeal. I'm glad times have changed because I have a strong inclination to eat food on a regular basis and whatever I eat, has to be worth it. If I am ingesting calories, it better taste good.

Sugar-free snacks are nasty. Don't pretend they are not. And, sugar-free does not mean carb-free. You have probably tasted them before—cardboard in consistency and incredibly tasteless. I have yet to find a single sugar-free food worth the calories, unless you are talking about well-done, crispy bacon and scrambled eggs with cheese, which are (almost) carb-free foods. I will knock you out of the way for those. Thank goodness my cholesterol remains in check! If I am going to eat something, I want to enjoy it, so I still indulge my sweet tooth daily with a treat or two. If there are homemade chocolate chip cookies around, I might even eat two at once (gasp!). Food is something to be appreciated and enjoyed, not feared and worrisome. If my sugar goes up, I'll be quick to get it down. I check my blood sugar sometimes up to a gazillion times a day to keep it all in check. That may seem slightly excessive and a gross exaggeration, but take into account that every time I get a strange high or low reading, I check it twice to make sure the number is accurate. I can't tell you how many times I have had false readings and treated myself accordingly. It's bad news to get a 304 blood sugar reading and give yourself six units of insulin when your blood sugar is *really* at 113. Try eating yourself out of that deficit! That's the one time that I do not enjoy food whatsoever.

The truth is, most people pay more attention to the gasoline they put in their cars than the food they put in their mouths. Diabetics need to be the exception. Food and eating do not have to be complicated, and at times, candy can be your sweetest friend. When you think of managing blood sugar, odds are you obsess over everything you can't have. Although it's certainly important to limit the no-no's (such as white, refined breads and pastas and fried, fatty, processed foods) that you shouldn't eat, it's just as crucial to pay attention to what you *should* eat. Let's start with that.

Power Foods

If you already follow a diet filled with whole grains, fresh fruits, veggies, and lean protein, congratulations! You are on your way to a long and healthy life and taking tight control over your weight and blood sugar levels. For those who are taking baby steps toward eating better, this list of *power foods* will help you on your way. Numerous nutrition and diabetes experts singled out the following power foods because they're packed with the four healthy nutrients (fiber, omega-3s, calcium, and vitamin D) and are exceptionally versatile, so you can use them in recipes, as add-ons to meals, or as stand-alone snacks. These foods are commanding enough to help lower your cholesterol, reduce your risk of heart disease and cancer, keep blood sugar levels stable, and put you in a better mood. All of these foods are real, unprocessed foods. You will not find corn chips or marshmallows in any power food category.

1. Beans

Beans, beans the magical fruit. Beans provide a lot more than just a good passing-gas joke. They are high in fiber (which helps you to feel fuller, longer); they help to steady your blood sugar; and they even lower cholesterol so that you can eat more bacon.

(I'm joking.) They're also a not-too-shabby source of calcium, a mineral that research shows can help burn body fat. Beans are loaded with protein, and unlike other proteins we commonly eat (think cow), beans are low in saturated fat. That's a good thing because you don't want to gunk up your arteries and get heart disease, do you?

2. Dairy

You're not going to find a better source of calcium and vitamin D—a potent diabetes-quelling combination—than in dairy foods such as milk, cottage cheese, and yogurt. One study found that women who consumed more than twelve hundred milligrams of calcium and more than eight hundred international units (IU) of vitamin D a day were 33 percent less likely to develop diabetes than those taking in less of both nutrients. That study means nothing to me; I used to drink a ton of milk growing up and still have diabetes, but hey, if it works for some, that's great!

You can get calcium and vitamin D from other foods as well, but none combine them like dairy does. Stick to fat-free or low-fat versions of your favorite dairy foods—"regular" has tons of saturated fat. Translation: You will gain weight and you will destroy your arteries.

Drink skim milk with some meals instead of soda or juice. Soda and juice are just empty calories. Eliminate them or save them to raise your blood glucose levels when you are sick of eating glucose tablets. You can also add in yogurt or cottage cheese as a snack or dessert. In your supermarket, there are some super-yummy low-fat Greek yogurts (which contain twice the protein of regular yogurt) that have side mixers of granola, flax, fruit, chia seeds, and dark chocolate.

3. Salmon

I love salmon, and nutritionists can't recommend this seriously healthy fish enough. It's a rich source of omega-3 fatty acids, which are healthy fats that reduce the risk of heart disease, whittle your waistline, reduce inflammation, help with memory loss, and improve insulin resistance. Salmon is also one of the best nondairy sources of vitamin D around. Plus, don't you remember Grandma saying that salmon is brain food?

4. Tuna

Another amazingly healthy fish, tuna, also contains omega-3s and a respectable amount of vitamin D, to boot. Eat it in moderation though because tuna can be high in mercury, a compound that may cause neurological problems in huge doses. You don't want to mess around with that. You've got enough on your plate already.

5. Barley

One of the healthiest grains you're probably not eating, barley is rich in soluble fibers that lowers cholesterol and helps control blood sugar. Thanks to its fiber abundance, barley can also help steady your blood sugar while filling you up—a weight-loss bonus. The grain even boasts a modest amount of calcium. It's not the easiest thing to add into your diet, but it is well worth it.

6. Oats

There's nothing more comforting than a warm bowl of oatmeal in the morning. Like barley and beans, oats are a diabetes power food because of their fiber content—fiber is good, people! Research shows that oat lovers can also lower total and "bad" LDL cholesterol and improve insulin resistance. I'm sure you know this information from watching the Quaker Oats commercials. What you might not know, however, is that all the soluble fiber that oats contain slows the rate at which your body can break down and absorb carbohydrates, which means that your blood sugar levels stay stable. A stable blood sugar equals a happy diabetic.

They say that breakfast is the most important meal of the day, and the easiest way to eat oats is straight from your cereal bowl. Taking insulin and eating a healthy breakfast are the two best things you can do to combat dawn phenomenon, and a high-fiber, high-protein meal will do just that. You can also sneak oats into all kinds of recipes—from pancakes to meatloaf to cookies. Oatmeal chocolate chip, anyone?

7. Berries

Berries are nature's candy, but unlike sugary confections from the checkout aisle, they're loaded with fiber and antioxidants called *polyphenols.* The darker the berry, the more antioxidants they have. That means that they are good for your ticker. They also improve memory by protecting your brain from inflammation and boosting communication between brain cells.

Delectable on their own, berries are also extra flavorful when stirred into oatmeal, ice cream, or even salads. Fresh berries freeze well, so if you're not going to eat them right away, store them in your freezer so that you always have some on hand.

8. Greens

You're probably thinking of lettuce, and I don't want to disappoint, but we are talking about collard greens, a staple of Southern cooking. This category of veggie is incredibly diverse, with choices such as turnip, mustard, and beet greens as well as chard. All are outstanding sources of Vitamin K, fiber, and calcium. Greens may also be good for your heart, thanks to the folate they contain. This B vitamin appears to lower levels of homocysteine, an amino acid that in high amounts can raise heart disease risk. Greens are kind of bitter, and many people consider them an acquired taste, but when prepared well, they are de-lish!

9. Lentils

Like their bean cousins, lentils are loaded with fiber. If you're not a meat person, lentils are a good alternative source of meat-free protein; they also contain a variety of vitamins and minerals. When given lentil as a soup option, always choose it—tasty and good for you!

10. Flaxseed

These tiny seeds of the flax plant pack a big health punch. Not only is flaxseed loaded with plant omega-3s but it also has more lignans (compounds that may prevent endometrial and ovarian cancer) than any other food. In several large studies, researchers have found a link between increased ALA intake and lower odds of heart disease, heart attack, and other cardiovascular issues. These magic seeds also show promise for lowering cholesterol and have been shown to be effective in lowering A1C levels of type 2 diabetics.

Add ground flaxseed to all kinds of food, such as oatmeal, low-fat cottage cheese, and fruit smoothies. I sprinkle it on almost anything. Keep it in the refrigerator to get the best taste and to have it last the longest.

11. Peanut Butter

Who doesn't like peanut butter? Believe it or not, peanut butter has been linked to reduced diabetes risk. The fiber content may have something to do with it, and because this classic comfort food contains mostly monounsaturated fat, it's considered heart healthy. The calories are on the high side, however, so pay attention to the serving size. Eat it alone or on apples, whole-grain waffles, bananas—pretty much anything!

12. Dark Chocolate

Saving the best for last. Rich in antioxidant flavonoids, this deceptively decadent sweet may help improve your good and bad cholesterol and reduce your blood pressure. One ounce contains about 145 calories, 15g of carbs and 9 grams of fat, so nibble just a little—every day. It will make you happy.

Food For Thought

Our good-for-you food list would not be complete without mentioning the following extra healthy foods that are among the best for diabetics:

- An *apple* a day *does* help to keep the doctor away, especially the cardiologist.

- *Asparagus* has tons of vitamin K and is a natural diuretic, although it does make your pee smell funky.

- *Avocados* are known for their heart-healthy fat, which keeps you satisfied while helping to absorb other nutrients.

- *Broccoli* is rich in vitamin C and beta-carotene, which helps the body to produce Vitamin A, which promotes healthy vision, teeth, bones, and skin.

- *Carrots* are great raw or cooked and are rich in beta-carotene, which lowers the risk of developing type 2 diabetes in people with a genetic disposition for the disease. Plus, they are good for your eyesight, mainly night vision. As my dad always said as I was growing up, "Eat your carrots; they are good for your eyes. Have you ever seen a rabbit wearing glasses?"

- Add *garlic* to almost anything, and it tastes that much better; plus, it has been shown to have many healthful benefits, including lowering blood pressure and cholesterol.

- *Kale* is increasing in popularity and is tasty, nutritious, and highly versatile in the kitchen. Plus, it too reduces the risk of developing type 2 diabetes.

- When craving something sweet, try some *melon.* Watermelon, cantaloupe, and honeydew all are bursting with nutrients, are low in calories, and taste delicious.

- *Nuts* are one of the healthiest food choices you can make. They contain a superabundance of heart-healthy substances and can even improve blood sugar control. Just watch out because they are high in calories.

- The mild, nutty grain *quinoa* (pronounced KEEN-wah) contains all nine essential amino acids, making it a complete protein. It prevents blood sugar spikes and staves off hunger.

- Sweet and juicy, *red grapefruit* helps to decrease bad cholesterol and lower blood pressure. This delicious orb packs tons of fiber and antioxidant power.

- *Red peppers* are actually green peppers that have been allowed to ripen on the vine longer while they load up with a gaggle of good-for-you nutrients. Look for ways to mix them into your diet.

- *Oysters* keep your immune system strong and provide a quarter of your daily iron per serving; plus, they provide all the zinc you need for an entire day. Not to mention, oysters also have a reputation for inspiring passion if you need some more of that in your life.

- *Soy* is a high quality protein and a fantastic source of niacin, folate, zinc, potassium, iron, and alpha-linolenic acid, plus it's high in fiber, and there is no shortage of soy products available on the market today.

- Popeye was right, *spinach* is good for you. Just a half cup of this low-calorie, leafy green veggie provides more than five times your daily dose of Vitamin K, plus loads of folate and vitamin C.

- *Tea* (green or black) reduces the risk of heart disease, improves cholesterol levels, alleviates stress, and reduces the risk of cancer. Plus, it has the added benefit of hydrating you throughout the day.

- *Tomatoes* are loaded with lycopene, which makes your skin look younger and keeps your heart healthy.

- A glass or two of *acai juice* can dramatically boost the amount of antioxidants in your blood. Beware it is high in carbs though.

- *Grapes* are a leading source of resveratrol, the plant chemical responsible for the heart-healthy benefits of red wine. You could also drink some red wine too. *Salud!*

Unfortunately, none of these foods prevent a person from developing type 1, but they do help to keep you healthy!

Do you speak any other languages besides English? I do. I speak Italian, Spanish, and *Carbonese*. What's Carbonese, you ask? No, it's not the language of the great country of Carbon; rather, it's the language of carbohydrate counting. With diabetes, you enter a whole different world and culture, and you can't just eat whatever you want there. You have to learn the language, and you can't just be "good" at it—you have to be great. It's one of the most effective ways of properly managing your blood sugars and well worth the effort to learn, considering the impact it has on your life.

More than 90 percent of the carbs derived from starches and sugars end up as glucose that moves through the blood to your cells. Half of the day's insulin is used to balance the carbohydrate that we eat in foods. The other half meets the background insulin we need, and this need remains relatively steady from day to day.

So, what are these carbs we talk about so much, anyway? The dictionary describes them as any of a large group of organic compounds occurring in foods and living tissues, including sugars, starch, and cellulose. They contain hydrogen and oxygen in the same ratio as water (two to one) and typically can be broken down to release energy in the animal body. That's the scientific definition of a carbohydrate, but we know them best as anything that tastes good.

You find carbs in:

- Grains (breads, pasta, cereals)

- Fruits (one serving averaging about 15 carbs)

- Vegetables (some are more starchier than others)

- Root crops (potatoes, sweet potatoes, and yams)

- Beer, wine, and some hard liquors

- Desserts and candies

- Most milk products, except cheese

- Foods that end in -ose, such as sucrose, fructose, maltose

In a healthy diet, most carbohydrates would come from nutrient-dense foods. Nutrient-dense foods and complex carbs—such as whole grains, fruits, legumes, vegetables, nonfat or low-fat milk, and yogurt—contain a high volume of vitamins, minerals, fiber, and protein in proportion to their calorie content. These micro-ingredients allow glucose to be processed correctly and present the development of deficiencies that generate "carb craving." They also tend to be lower on the glycemic index. The glycemic index is a measure of how quickly blood glucose levels rise after eating a particular food.

Foods high on the glycemic index include white bread, white rice, cereals, potato, candy, bagels, dates and pretzels. Foods lower on the index include beans, seeds, grains, yogurt, vegetables and some fruits. Ice cream, bananas, popcorn, tacos, and macaroni and cheese fall somewhere in the middle. A smart approach for any person, with or without diabetes, is to stay away from foods with high glycemic levels. Repeated blood sugar spikes stress the organs that make up the metabolic engine of your body. If you stop living large and back off the high-impact glycemics, the longer your body will function normally. Sugar isn't responsible for all of the world's problems, just most of them.

Low-nutrient foods, such as candy and regular sodas, contain carbohydrates but lack the other nutrients your cells require for health. Because they contain simple sugar or refined grains, they are high on the glycemic index and are more likely to cause the blood sugar to spike. Cue the drama button here. They may be eaten in small amounts, but nutrient-dense foods such as brown rice and broccoli are better for both your health and your blood sugars.

You measure carbohydrates in grams, which are a unit of weight like pounds or ounces. Because of their very small size (it takes twenty-eight grams to equal a single ounce), grams can be used to accurately measure carbohydrate. Simply weighing foods does not tell you how much carbohydrate they contain, because most foods are not purely carbohydrate. For example, even though 224 grams (one cup) of milk, a 160-gram slice of watermelon, a fourteen-gram rectangular graham cracker (two squares), and twelve grams (one tablespoon) of sugar have different weights, they all contain exactly twelve grams of carbohydrate and require the same carb bolus to cover them. The milk and watermelon contain water, whereas graham crackers have other ingredients. Only a few foods such as table sugar and lollipops contain entirely carbohydrates, so their weight on a gram scale will be exactly the same as the number of grams of carbohydrate they contain.

Knowing a food's weight and the percentage of its weight that is composed of carbohydrate allows for precise measurement. Knowing your carb factor, which is how many carbs are covered by one unit of insulin, allows precise insulin dosing. Your carb factor is a personal measurement; only you can figure out your factor (with your doctor's help), and it usually involves trial and error. If you feel like comparing, my current carb ratio is 1:6 at breakfast, 1:12 at lunch and 1:14 at dinner.

The carb content of almost every food you can think of can be determined by food labels, online sites (there are many), phone applications, a scale, and a list of carb factors. All the required information is at your fingertips. Coincidentally, that is exactly where you draw your glucose tests from.

Like any new skill, counting grams of carbohydrates will take a couple of months, maybe even longer, to master. As time passes, you will train your eye to estimate accurately both serving sizes and weights, whether eating out or at home. Carbohydrate in the food we eat has the greatest impact on our blood sugars. Balancing carbs with insulin lets you keep your blood sugars controlled, and carb counting is an important tool for doing this. Start reading, speak to a nutritionist if you can, and have your Smartphone handy to look a food up on a moment's notice. It will make your diabetes so much easier to manage.

Exercise

Carb counting and nutrition go arm in arm with exercise, and it would be a great omission not to bring that up next. Here is all you have to know: You need to exercise every day. There's no need for a crazy workout; just get your walk on! If you want variety, then play tennis, golf, run, jog, play soccer or baseball, have relay races in the backyard with the kids, hike, skip, hop, jump rope, take ballet or Pilates, learn kickboxing or karate, get a trainer, lift weights, do jumping jacks or sit-ups or push-ups, ride a bike, go bowling, climb rocks, dance, fly a kite, swim, canoe, ski, or twirl a baton. Just get up off of your butt, get the blood pumping, and *do something.*

If you need to know why you absolutely need to exercise, here's the laundry list:

- It will lower your blood glucose and your blood pressure.

- It will lower your bad cholesterol and raise your good cholesterol.

- It will improve your body's ability to use insulin.

- It will lower your risk for heart disease and stroke.

- It will keep your heart and bones strong.

- It will keep your joints flexible.

- It will lower your risk of falling.

- It will help you lose weight.

- It will reduce your body fat.

- It will give you more energy.

- It will reduce your stress levels.

If you need additional reasons that are a little more vain, your clothing will fit better and you will look much better naked.

Along with exercise, you can incorporate extra movement into your daily activities. This increases the number of calories you burn. Here are some easy examples:

- Walk around while you talk on the phone.

- Play with the kids.

- Take the dog for a walk.

- Get up to change the TV channel instead of using the remote control.

- Work in the garden or rake leaves.

- Clean the house, or even a closet. You'll be happy you did.

- Wash the car.

- Stretch out your chores. For example, make two trips to take the laundry downstairs instead of one.

- Park at the far end of the shopping center parking lot and walk to the store. You car will have fewer dings in it as well.

- At the grocery store, walk every aisle. You might even leave the store without forgetting something. Although do not do this when you are hungry, because it may make you buy more!

- At work, walk over to see a coworker instead of calling or emailing. Face-to-face contact is refreshing and more genuine.

- Take the stairs instead of the elevator.

- Stretch or walk around instead of taking a coffee break and eating.

- During your lunch break, walk to the post office or do other errands.

If I've learned one thing in life, it's that there are always exceptions to everything. If you have diabetes complications, some kinds of exercise can make your problems worse. For example, activities that increase the pressure in the blood vessels of your eyes, such as lifting heavy weights, can make diabetic eye problems worse. If nerve damage from diabetes has made your feet numb, your doctor may suggest that you try swimming instead of walking for aerobic exercise.

If you have type 1 diabetes, avoid strenuous exercise when you have ketones in your blood or urine. Ketones are chemicals your body might make when your blood glucose level is too high and your insulin level is too low. Too many ketones can make you sick. If you exercise when you have ketones in your blood or urine, your blood glucose level may go even higher.

If you have type 2 diabetes and your blood glucose is high but you don't have ketones, light or moderate exercise will probably lower your blood glucose. Ask your health care team whether you should exercise when your blood glucose is high. .

If you have numb feet, you might not feel pain in them. Blisters from exercise might get worse because you don't notice them. Without proper care, minor foot problems can turn into serious conditions (which I swore I would not bring up in this book). Make sure you exercise in cotton socks and comfortable, well-fitting shoes designed for the activity you are doing. After you exercise, check your feet for cuts, sores, bumps, or redness. Call your doctor if any foot problems develop.

Physical activity can also cause low blood glucose. Low blood glucose can happen while you exercise, right afterward, or even up to a day later. It can make you feel shaky, weak, confused, grumpy, hungry, or tired. You may sweat a lot or get a headache or even pass out. If you check your blood sugar often, however, you can reduce the chances of that happening or can head off lows (and highs) before they get too bad. Testing your blood sugar frequently is one of the smartest preventative measures you can take when you are living with diabetes. It takes considerable effort, but glucose levels will never get too out of control if you are keeping them constantly in check. So please, test, test, test!

Another thing to consider when beginning an exercise program is decreasing insulin that peaks before exercise so you do't go down to low in the middle of your workout. You might also decrease basal insulin at night if you exercised a lot during the day, or eat extra carbs at the time you begin to exercise, depending on how intense you plan on working out. Your doctor can figure out the best plan of action for your new fitness plan. Don't let diabetes stop you from being fit, healthy and having a rockin' bod.

I have one last issue to address in this chapter. It has been found that a number of young people with type 1 diabetes have used their disease as a weight loss method similar to bulimia, but worse. Instead of throwing up to lose weight, a diabetic lets his or her blood sugars run purposely high, keeping constant ketones in the body and causing the body to eat itself. The term the diabetic community has given this disease is *diabulimia.* If you think any diabetic person you know might have an issue with body image or weight, please get him or her professional help quickly. This is double jeopardy to one's health.

Chapter Ten

I'm Not Diabetic; I'm Pancreatically Challenged

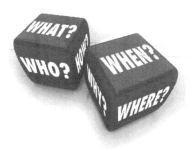

I've never been a huge game show fan, but one night I dreamt that I was a contestant on the show *Family Feud*. I was up at the podium, and the qualifying question was presented to me: "The top six answers are on the board. We surveyed 100 people with the following question: *What is the first thing you do in the morning upon waking?*" I buzzed in first and answered, "Test my blood!" As you can probably imagine, that was not even close to being in the top 100. "Go to the bathroom," "Brush my teeth," and "Check my phone" scored considerably higher. I lost. What a bummer.

That dream shows just how different those of us with diabetes are from anyone else out there. We have a unique way of going about our days and our lives. Even our dreams sometimes revolve around being diabetic. Before I move from my cozy little nest of a bed, I test my blood glucose. Then I start my day accordingly. Some days it might be with a shot, other days with some grapefruit juice. Sometimes an anomaly might even occur, and I am able to hop straight into the shower.

What it comes down to is that no matter what you are doing, where you are, how you feel, who you are with, what time zone you are in, how tired you are, how busy you are, or how emotionally drained you are, you have to think about the fact that you have diabetes.

Every day the same questions run through my head:

Where is my meter? I cannot even begin to tell you how many times I have lost that damn thing and have had to backtrack through my day to find it. I've lost it at Target, at concerts, in my car, in parking lots, even in my own bedroom. You name it, that pesky little thing has disappeared on me at least a hundred times over the years. I've even been thrown into a full-blown panic attack, more than once, over not being able to find it. I just might invent a tracking device for it. I certainly can't imagine I'm the only one this happens to! Is there an app for that?

Do I have enough test strips with me for the day? I've run out of those oodles of times too. Then the guessing game begins. For some reason it's always when I am out to dinner or with friends, casually eating and drinking whatever I want. That gets curtailed quite a bit when I realize I have an empty strip container with me. Curses! Either the fun comes to an abrupt end or I gamble and try to guess what my blood sugar is. This is never, ever a good move, and I've rarely been right.

I've come to realize my whole world depends on this little tiny machine. I'm so attached to it that I do not even go for a walk around the block without it. It's my life line. Thank goodness for technology, though; a century ago, none of us stood a chance of gracing this Earth much past our thirtieth birthdays.

Have I forgotten any of my other supplies? When I am packing for vacation you would think one thing that I would always remember would be my insulin, natch. Admittedly, I have forgotten it a handful of times. It's never fun to call your doctor at midnight from another country to have him call in a prescription for you to a random pharmacy. I once stayed at a hotel uptown in New York City and traveled all the way downtown to a restaurant in Tribeca, forgetting my shot in my hotel room. That wasn't fun, wasting half of the night in cabs and half of my martini money for fare. Not to mention obsessing about the high blood sugar that caused me to look for the insulin to begin with!

How many carbs are in this food I am eating? Eating out in a restaurant or eating something without a carbohydrate listing on the side of the packaging will inevitably always throw me off course. It's next to impossible to know how much of any ingredient is in homemade food. Apart from that, I'd like to think I can count the carbs in every other food type there is. I am a human carb-counting machine. The only restaurants, and I use that term loosely, that can provide you with the amount of carbohydrates contained in their food on neat little nutritional trifold charts are the places that aren't very nutritional at all, for example, McDonald's, Wendy's, and Chick-Fil-A. Although those little charts and fast food places came in handy when I was pregnant and craving a Taco Bell chalupa.

Through life coaching, I have been helping individuals improve their lives in areas such as overall life transformation, health and fitness, and confidence building. I always suggest to clients who want to lose weight to follow what I fondly refer to as the "diabetic diet." If you can count carbs and not exceed a certain amount suited for your body type, you will lose weight. It's that simple. I have remained close to the same weight since high school. (Don't hate me, but I have always wanted to say that and finally have the opportunity!) The only other thing you need to do, along with counting carbs, is exercise. Yes, I'm taking every opportunity I can to repeat this over and over. Try to work in at least forty-five minutes a day, four or five days a week. Run, walk, swim, even skip if you enjoy it, just get up and do something!

Is anybody watching me test my blood? Do they wonder what I am doing? I was slightly disturbed by what happened to me at a Las Vegas casino a few years back. I love gambling. Probably too much. I was playing Texas hold 'em at one of the tables, and I pulled out my blood meter on my lap and tested my blood. I threw it back into my handbag and within mere seconds I was tapped on the shoulder by two men in suits who politely asked me to get up and come with them. Although oddly flattered, I told them I was not an escort and to leave me alone. Then they *demanded* I come with them, flashed a badge at me, and I got up and went. They took me into a back room off of the casino floor and asked me to show them the contents of my purse. I insisted to know what this was about. They told me that I was observed on video using some sort of device that led them to believe I was card counting. I kid you not. We all got a good laugh when I showed them my blood meter, but I felt violated in so many ways. Not to mention that I was wearing a skirt and don't think I had my legs completely closed while sitting in my seat. I'm sure the cameras got a spectacular view of that too. I got a quick apology and was sent on my merry way. I was hoping for some chip compensation for embarrassing me and making me look like a common criminal, but that wasn't in the cards (pun intended).

I need more supplies. Do I have enough money in my checking account to cover them today? Diabetes is an expensive condition. My heart goes out to those with diabetes who cannot afford health insurance. While I am entirely grateful to have health insurance considering so much of our world population is without it, I will say that health insurance is for healthy people, not for the people with diseases who need it the most.

When you are diabetic, you are constantly dealing with an unlimited source of frustration and grief. Health insurance companies will have you cursing, kicking, and screaming most of the time. I know their customer service teams are not responsible for the crappy insurance policies, and I do often apologize for flipping out on them when I do. However, I would love to get my hands on those policymakers, chief executive officers, and all the rest of the top dogs who come up with these asinine rules and regulations.

Wow. Where did all that come from? Well, my health insurance changed the other day, and when I went to pick up my insulin, it cost two hundred fifty dollars for a three-month supply. Excuse me?

Why is my blood glucose low? Why is it high? Why won't it come up? These questions are enough to make a sane person lose it, which means I do have a valid excuse most of the time.

Is this an accurate blood sugar reading?

So many times the blood sugar reading can be inaccurate on your meter - there is also a built in 10% variability to factor in on top of it. You feel low, but it reads normal or high. This has happened to me hundreds of times over the years. Not only does this waste a strip, but you have to prick yourself again. I have combated these inaccuracies by trying to use an alcohol swab on my finger, but sometimes it's just not possible, or I'm in a rush, or I'm just plain lazy.

Do I have a snack with me in my bag if my sugar drops?

I should just carry around an intravenous bag of glucose for the number of times my sugar drops when I am not at home. I have gone through a litany of products that I favor when it comes time for sugary snacks to raise my glucose levels. I can definitely credit Juicy Juice, Sprees, candy corn, Peeps, Sour Patch Kids, and CranGrape juice by Ocean Spray, as well as good old sour-apple glucose tablets with saving my life at one point or another. Most of the time I have quite the hypostash with me. Heaven forbid if my kids try to touch it. Sometimes I realize that when I'm in public place and I loudly exclaim to one of my sons to get their cute little hands off of mommy's juice boxes, I look like either the meanest mommy around or the craziest. I'm kind of okay with crazy, but I do not want to be looked at as Mommie Dearest.

Are my basal rates correct? Did I over bolus? Ah, the joys of pumping! The insulin pump is one of the greatest inventions in the history of diabetes. I loved it for a handful of years and then started despising it. I think it's good to mix it up a little bit and take a pumping holiday whenever you feel the need. I could no longer tolerate the tubing, the alarms, injecting the settings, sleeping with it, the fact that I had to have it hooked to me all day, and generally speaking, the sight of it. When I loved my precious pump, I loved it with a passion. My A1C levels were fantastic, the ease of use was uncontested, and the spontaneity it provided to let me eat whenever and wherever I pleased without pulling out a hypodermic needle was fantastic. I've gotten so many dirty looks over the years in restaurants. I just want to say to all of those people who have looked down on me and my syringe: *at least you don't have diabetes!* I think you will be okay seeing a needle for a second. If by chance you are one of those people who pass out from the sight of them, please try not to look at me.

I think it's amusing that when people see how *unnoticeable* your pump looks clipped to your waist, they exclaim, "Wow, it looks just like a beeper!" What is this, 1991? Who even uses a beeper anymore? Anyone who does use a beeper looks a bit uncool so think about that the next time someone tells you your pump looks like one.

Since I am on a roll about pumps, I have one more complaint. The pump companies insist that you can stick the device in your bra for safekeeping, and no one can see it. How come when I stick it in mine, I look like a freak of nature with a third breast? Very unattractive. I think this only works for women with big guns or excessive cleavage. I look deformed.

I was in the airport the other day and watched a woman get a full body scan and then a pat down because she had a pump in her bra. Transportation Security Administration officials and everyone else in the near vicinity watched her pull it out of her cleavage and start explaining why it was in there. I took one sympathetic glance and started walking to my gate, thinking I've been there before—explaining it to anyone who happened to get a gander at it, whether in the airport, the supermarket, a theme park, or a fitting room.

Did I take my bedtime shot? Sometimes I wonder if my memory is going, but then I remind myself how busy I am all day and night and how many directions I'm pulled in. If someone (namely one of my children) distracts me (which happens all day long), I forget if I gave myself my long-acting insulin dose at bedtime. That's not something you want to take twice. My next invention might be a solution to this dilemma.

My vision got blurry for a second, do I have retinopathy? My foot fell asleep, was I sitting on it wrong or do I have neuropathy? With diabetes comes constant concern for how the highs and lows have affected your body over time. I am going to refer to my friend Wiki (pedia) to help me define *diabetic retinopathy* and *neuropathy* in case you are interested. Here are the abridged versions:

> *Diabetic retinopathy:* Damage to the retina caused by complications of diabetes that can eventually lead to blindness. The good news is, you are in charge of preventing this from happening. Research indicates that many new cases could be reduced if the eyes were properly and vigilantly treated and monitored and blood sugar is controlled. The longer a person has diabetes, the higher his or her chances of developing diabetic retinopathy. Make sure you get your peepers checked yearly.

> *Diabetic neuropathy:* Damage to the nerves that causes loss of feeling to limbs and extremities. Your doctor can test for this with a vibrating tuning fork or a piece of monofilament touching your toes. You don't want neuropathy, and you can prevent it. Take care of yourself.

This leads me to a little ditty about my past life as a fashionista in New York City. Fashion Week in New York is the week that designers, editors, public relations people, and lovers of all things fabulous come together to carry on and to pull out all the stops when it comes time to getting dressed, being seated, and sipping champagne from little splits with straws. These crazy weeks all seem like a blur now, because back then I was always overtired and usually underdressed for the weather. It doesn't matter though, because they say fashion has no temperature (although I *have* always wondered who "they" were).

It was February, and I had been wearing a pair of pointy stiletto Christian Louboutins (those phenomenally sexy sky-high heels with the red soles) for three days straight. Those suckers were killing my feet. In the same way that I am on the side of the "fashion knows no temperature" crowd, I also come from the mindset that you have to suffer a little bit to look stunning, so the shoes remained on my feet all day as I walked from show to show and party to party. Research says that it is hard for the brain to remember pain, and that is why women have more than one baby, but I challenge you to find one woman who can't completely take herself back to a moment of shoe pain, whether it's from jamming her tootsies into shoes that are one size too small or walking all day in heels that are four inches too high.

Skip to a few days later, and I had my biannual visit to the endocrinologist scheduled. When he pulled out that little vibrating pitchfork and put it on my big toe to check for neuropathy in my feet, I couldn't feel a thing. This was highly concerning for him and a "holy crap!" moment for me. He decided to put me on a regimen of B12 shots to help fend off the possible nerve damage I had going on in my feet. The B12 shots are fantastic. I started referring to them as my "Superwoman shots" because they seemed to give me tons of energy and put me in a great mood. I didn't really need them; when my feet got some much needed rest in a pair of flip flops, the feeling came back to my toes. I kept getting the B12 shots, though. I'm slightly addicted to the way they make me feel. I know you probably don't want to take another shot if you really don't have to, but I'm telling you, I swear by these.

Even though the fashion industry is part of my past, champagne is still very much a part of my current life, as is an opulent bottle of Cabernet when the mood hits me. Let's face it, almost every diabetic person has probably had a drink or two or three or four. The American Diabetes Association tells us that alcohol is a toxin and that the diabetic's body reacts to alcohol like a poison, which makes me feel a little bad about all the poison I have ingested since turning twenty-one. However, the fact is, alcohol is socially acceptable and present at most events and gatherings. Like everything else, moderation is key. Too much of anything is never good for you. I am thankful that my diagnosis occurred after the crazy college years, but I do wish that it was caught earlier for so many obvious reasons.

Alcohol can induce low blood glucose levels. Typically, when glucose levels drop, the liver converts stored carbohydrate into glucose. If alcohol is consumed, the liver acts to clear that from the blood instead, but while it is busy processing alcohol, it stops releasing glucose. This glucose-lowering effect can last for as long as eight to twelve hours after drinking, especially if you have been drinking on an empty stomach or shortly after taking insulin or other glucose-lowering oral medications. Also, because it takes two hours for just one ounce of alcohol to metabolize and leave your system, the risk continues long after the glass is empty. The onset of hypoglycemia can occur very quickly and in severe cases can result in all those bad things I'm still not going to utter.

I've always wanted to do a study on the effects of alcohol on diabetes. I think a cure lies somewhere in that realm. My blood glucose always runs low the day after drinking, so there must be some connection. I've mentioned this to my doctor, and he asked me to promise him I wouldn't use my theory as a way to manage my blood sugar numbers. For the record, I wouldn't, and he knows that. He was just covering his ass.

Alcohol may be the hardest "food" for people with diabetes to manage because social drinking is so pervasive in our society (and so much fun)! If you are diabetic (and healthy), moderate drinking is acceptable provided that proper precautions are taken. For individuals with well-controlled diabetes, alcohol intake should follow guidelines that the USDA (US Department of Agriculture) has established for the general population: one drink for women and two for men, daily. An added precaution is to always eat something before you drink alcohol; you need the glucose from food because your liver will stop producing it once you drink alcohol.

Carefully check the level of what you're drinking and be sure to account for added calories and carbohydrates in fruit juices, sodas, and other mixers. Check the proof of distilled spirits and the alcohol level of beer and wines. Don't exercise before drinking; exercise lowers blood glucose levels, and drinking alcohol will reduce glucose further. Dancing counts as exercise, so think about skipping the drinks if you are hitting the dance floor. Be prepared for hypoglycemia in case your blood glucose levels dip below seventy, and be aware that glucagon will not help treat alcohol-induced hypoglycemia. Also, never treat hypoglycemia with a cocktail, even if it's a super sweet frozen strawberry daiquiri. Bring along your blood glucose monitor and check your levels frequently. Warn a friend or companion that you are diabetic and explain to them what to do in case of a hypoglycemic attack. This is important because hypoglycemia can resemble intoxication.

Please never drink to excess. It's not good for anyone, but it's especially not good for a diabetic.

We see how alcohol can affect your blood glucose considerably for both men and women. However, women have an additional factor that can cause dramatic swings in numbers. At first, you think you're just imagining it. You're going along and everything seems fine. You're in good spirits, eating well, getting regular workouts, and your blood glucose levels are on target most of the time. Then, for some unexplained reason, everything seems out of whack. Maybe your blood glucose levels are too high; maybe they're too low. Then you check the calendar. Oh, yeah—it's that time of the month.

If you have trouble keeping your blood glucose levels on target just before your period starts, you are not alone. Most women do. A survey of more than four hundred women revealed that nearly 70 percent experienced problems with blood glucose levels during their premenstrual period. The problem was more common among women who suffered from the moodiness associated with PMS.

A surefire cure to PMS is pregnancy. When I was identified as having type 1 diabetes and went from a carefree lifestyle to one of giving myself injections, monitoring what food I was eating, and hearing I might go blind, I was also told that if I did get pregnant one day it would be a high-risk pregnancy with no guarantees. That was twenty years ago and definitely not true today. Thanks to today's knowledge and technologies, women with both type 1 and type 2 diabetes can indeed have healthy children. I did.

That said, a woman's diabetes needs to be in good control before and throughout her pregnancy to safeguard her health and the healthiness of her baby. The key to a healthy pregnancy is good blood sugar control and prepregnancy planning. Experts recommend that a woman work with her obstetrician and an endocrinologist three to six months before conception so that her blood sugar levels, blood pressure level, cholesterol levels, and heart and vascular health are such that it's safe for her to be pregnant.

A fetus's heart, brain, nervous system, and other organs begin forming throughout the first five weeks of pregnancy, usually before a woman even knows she's pregnant. This initial phase of being pregnant poses risks, including birth defects and spontaneous abortion, so you have to take total control before you get knocked up, and you must abstain from alcohol as well. So enjoy your cocktails well in advance of considering getting preggo. Cheers!

Chapter Eleven

The Rich, Famous, and Really Smart Are Not Exempt

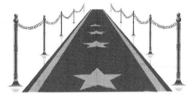

Diabetes should never stop someone from pursuing a dream, whether it's to become a well-known author, a world-renowned athlete, a glamorous Hollywood actress, or anything in between. Just when you thought you were all alone, you found me *and* all of these celebrated folks. Some are alive and some have passed on, but they all have shared in what you deal with every day. I'm kind of glad we have a Jonas Brother and Bret Michaels (he's my favorite) to supplement the list. I certainly do not wish this disease on anyone, but they speak out about having it and do not pretend it doesn't exist nor look at it as a weakness.

Entertainers

Jack Benny—comedian, actor (*The Jack Benny Program*), radio and television personality

Halle Berry—actress (*Monster's Ball, X-Men, Die Another Day*)

Wilford Brimley—actor (*Cocoon, The China Syndrome*)

J. Anthony Brown—actor (*Drumline*), comedian, radio personality, dLifeTV co-host

Delta Burke—actress (*Designing Women*), beauty pageant winner (Miss Florida, Miss USA)

James Cagney—actor (*Public Enemy, Angels With Dirty Faces, Yankee Doodle Dandy*)

Drew Carey—actor (*The Drew Carey Show*), comedian, game show host (*The Price Is Right*)

Nell Carter—actress (*Gimme a Break*)

Carol Channing—Broadway singer, actress (*The Carol Channing Show*)

Alvin Childress—actor (*Amos & Andy*)

Too Sweet

Dick Clark—television host (*American Bandstand*), producer, actor

James Doohan—actor (Scotty from *Star Trek*)

Dale Evans—actress (*The Yellow Rose of Texas, The Roy Rogers and Dale Evans Show*)

Don Francisco—television personality (*Sabado Gigante*)

Stephen Furst—actor (*Animal House*)

Victor Garber—actor (*Alias, Titanic, First Wives Club, Sleepless in Seattle*)

Jackie Gleason—actor (*The Honeymooners, Smokey and the Bandit, The Hustler*), comedian

Damon Dash—actor, producer, businessman (Roc-A-Fella Records)

Dorian Gregory—actor (*Baywatch Nights, Charmed, The Other Half*)

Tom Hanks—actor (*Big, Forrest Gump, Apollo 13, Saving Private Ryan, Cast Away, Toy Story*)

Dana Hill—actress (*Shoot the Moon, European Vacation*)

Larry King—talk show host

Al Lewis—actor (*The Munsters*)

Jerry Lewis—comedian, actor (*The Nutty Professor*), producer, director, writer, singer

Jerry Mathers—actor (*Leave it to Beaver*)

Mary Tyler Moore—actress (*Dick Van Dyke Show, Mary Tyler Moore Show, Ordinary People*), huge diabetes advocate

Tracy Morgan - comedian, actor (*30 Rock*)

Mother Love—entertainer, author, motivational speaker, dLifeTV CO-host

Richard Mulligan—actor (*Soap, Empty Nest*)

Carroll O'Conner—actor (*All in the Family, Heat of the Night*)

Park Overall—actress (*Empty Nest*)

Elizabeth Perkins—actress (*Big, Weeds*)

Della Reese—actress (*Touched by an Angel*), vocalist

Esther Rolle—actress (*Good Times*)

Sherri Shepherd—actress (*30 Rock*), television host (*The View*), comedian

Jean Smart—actress (*Designing Women, Sweet Home Alabama*)

Paul Sorvino—actor (*Goodfellas, Law & Order*), opera singer

Elaine Stritch—comedian, actress (*30 Rock*)

Spencer Tracy—actor (*Guess Who's Coming to Dinner*)

Jim Turner—actor (*Arli$$, Bewitched*), dLifeTV co-host

Aida Turturro—actress (*The Sopranos*)

Ben Vereen—actor (*Roots, Star Trek: The Next Generation*), performer, vocalist, humanitarian

Mae West—actress (*My Little Chickadee, I'm No Angel*)

Jane Wyman—actress (*The Yearling, Johnny Belinda, Falcon Crest*)

Athletes

Wasim Akram—Pakistani cricket fast bowler

Arthur Ashe —tennis player (Wimbledon winner)

Walter Barnes—football player (Philadelphia Eagles), actor

Sarah Bina—championship clogger

Ayden Byle—runner (first insulin-dependent man to run 6521.5 kilometers across North America)

Nick Boynton—ice hockey player (Boston Bruins)

Doug Burns—fitness consultant, record-holding strength athlete

Sean Busby—champion snowboarder

Bobby Clarke—ice hockey player (Philadelphia Flyers)

Ty Cobb—baseball player (Detroit Tigers)

Scott Coleman—swimmer (first man with diabetes to swim the English Channel, August 17, 1996)

Jay Cutler—football player (Chicago Bears)

Chris Dudley—basketball player (New York Knicks)

James "Buster" Douglas—heavyweight boxer

Kenny Duckett—football player (New Orleans Saints)

Rick Dudley—ice hockey assistant general manager (Montreal Canadiens), player

Scott Dunton—world-class surfer

Mike Echols—football player (Tennessee Titans)

Pam Fernandes—paralympic cyclist

Missy Foy—professional marathon runner

Curt Frasier—ice hockey player (Chicago Blackhawks)

Walt Frazier—basketball player (New York Knicks)

"Smokin' Joe" Frazier—boxer

Kris Freeman—cross-country skier (Olympics and National Championship)

Joe Gibbs—football coach (Washington Redskins)

Jorge "Giant" Gonzalez—professional wrestler, Argentinian basketball player, actor

Bill Gullickson—baseball player (Cincinnati Reds)

Gary Hall Jr.—swimmer (US Olympic gold medalist)

Jonathan Hayes—football player (Pittsburgh Steelers, Kansas City Chiefs)

Jay Hewitt—Ironman triathlete

Dave Hollins—baseball player (Philadelphia Phillies, 1993 World Series winners)

James "Catfish" Hunter—baseball player (New York Yankees Hall-of-Famer)

Too Sweet

Chuck Heidenrich—skier

Chris Jarvis—Canadian rower (world champion)

Jason Johnson—baseball player (Cleveland Indians)

Kelli Keuhne—golfer (LPGA)

Billie Jean King—tennis player

Jay Leeuwenburg—football player (Indianapolis Colts)

Mark Lowe—baseball player (Tampa Bay Rays)

Michael Earl Malone—son of former basketball player Moses Malone

Robert "Gorilla Monsoon" Marella—professional wrestler and commentator

Michelle McGann—golfer (LPGA)

Adam Morrison—basketball player (Gonzaga University)

Brandon Morrow—baseball player (Seattle Mariners)

David Pember—baseball player (Milwaukee Brewers)

Toby Petersen—ice hockey player (Pittsburgh Penguins, Dallas Stars)

Sir Steven Redgrave—rower (winner of five consecutive Olympic gold medals)

Ryan Reed—NASCAR driver

Dan Reichert—baseball player (Kansas City Royals)

Ham Richardson—tennis player

Jackie Robinson—baseball player (first African-American to play in Major League Baseball)

Sugar Ray Robinson—boxer

Ron Santo—baseball player (Chicago Cubs)

Mike Sinclair—football player (Philadelphia Eagles)

Kendall Simmons—football player (Pittsburgh Steelers)

Ron Springs—football player (Dallas Cowboys)

Jerry Stackhouse—basketball player (Dallas Mavericks)

Hank Stram—football coach (Kansas City Chiefs)

Bradley Suttle—baseball player (Texas Longhorns)

Bill Talbert—tennis player (Hall of Fame)

Jack Tatum—football player (Oakland Raiders, "The Assassin")

Sherri Turner—golfer (LPGA)

Scott Verplank—golfer (PGA)

Jo Ann Washam—golfer (LPGA)

David "Boomer" Wells—baseball player (San Diego Padres)

Dominique Wilkins—basketball player (Atlanta Hawks)

Wade Wilson—football quarterback coach (Dallas Cowboys), player (Oakland Raiders)

Dmitri Young—baseball player (Detroit Tigers, Washington Nationals)

Business People

James Conkling—*Founder, National Academy Recording Arts and Sciences, helped in the creation of the Grammy Award*

Bill and John Davidson—heads of Harley-Davidson Motorcycles

Tom Foster—former head of Foster Poultry Farms, one of the nation's top privately held companies

W.L. Gherra—board member, Payless Drugs

Ray Kroc—founder of McDonald's

Larry H. Miller—entrepreneur, owner of Utah Jazz

Paula Deen—celebrity chef

Politicians and World Leaders

Yuri Andropov—Soviet premier

President Hafez al-Assad—president of Syria

Menachem Begin—prime minister of Israel

Marion Barry—former mayor of Washington, D.C.

Samuel Block—civil rights activist

Ralph Bunche—Nobel Prize winner, United Nations diplomat

Paddy Devlin—Cofounder of the Social Democrat and Labor party in Northern Ireland

King Fahd—king of Saudi Arabia

Mikhail Gorbachev—general secretary of the Soviet Union

Mike Huckabee—Arkansas governor

Bill Janklow—former South Dakota governor and US representative

Wei Jingsheng—Chinese dissident

Joseph Kolter—US representative (Pennsylvania)

Nikita Kruschev—Soviet premier

Fiorello LaGuardia—former mayor of New York City

James Lloyd—US Congressman (California)

Winnie Mandela—South African anti-apartheid leader

Brian Mulroney—former prime minister

Gamal Abdel-Nasser—former leader of Egypt

Buddy Roemer—former governor of Louisiana and US representative

Anwar Sadat—president of Egypt

Sonia Sotomayor—associate justice of the US Supreme Court

Artists

Paul Cezanne—artist, painter

Sergey Ermakov—fashion designer

Suzanne Gardner—painter

Zippora Karz—ballet teacher, former NYC Ballet soloist

Walt Kelly—writer, illustrator, artist (*Pogo* comic)

Giacomo Puccini—operatic composer

Richard Bartlett—screenwriter

David Broder—columnist, *The Washington Post* (Pulitzer Prize winner)

Bryan Busby—chief meteorologist, KMBC (Kansas City, Missouri)

Fran Carpentier—editor, *Parade Magazine*

Sylvia Chase—journalist (*20/20*)

Rodolfo Garcia—reporter, Associated Press

Linda Goodman—author (*Linda Goodman's Sun Signs*)

Jim Hamblin—California news reporter

Ernest Hemingway—author (*For Whom the Bell Tolls, A Farewell to Arms, The Sun Also Rises*)

Phebe Robinson Jacobsen—archivist (worked with Alex Haley on *Roots*)

Nicole Johnson—author, diabetes advocate, dLifeTV CO-host, Miss America 1999

Ken Kesey—novelist (*One Flew Over The Cuckoo's Nest*)

Laura Kronen—Me!

Lyle Leverich—biographer

Maria Marin—international speaker, columnist, author and radio personality

Chris Matthews—political commentator, news anchor

Steve McCaffery—Canadian author, poet

Connie Pirner—teaching consultant for National Geographic

Mario Puzo—author (*The Godfather*)

Anne Rice—author (*Interview With a Vampire*)

Carl Rowan—nationally syndicated columnist and author

H. G. Wells—author (*War of the Worlds, The Time Machine, The Invisible Man*), founded the British Diabetic Association

Laura Ingalls Wilder—author (*Little House on the Prairie*)

Musicians

Nat Adderley—jazz musician

Ray Anderson—jazz musician

Syd Barret—singer (Pink Floyd)

Tony Bennett—jazz singer

Crystal Bowersox—folk-rock musician, *American Idol* contestant

Danny Joe Brown—member of Molly Hatchet

James Brown—musician ("The Godfather of Soul")

Johnny Cash—musician ("The Man in Black")

Bobby Charles—singer-songwriter

Mark Collie—country singer

David Crosby—member of Crosby, Stills, and Nash

Miles Davis—jazz musician

Johnny Darrell—country music singer

Phife Dawg—member of A Tribe Called Quest

Priscilla "P-Star" Diaz—entertainer, musician, and actress

Bo Diddley—singer

Mama Cass Elliott—member of The Mamas and the Papas

Ella Fitzgerald—singer

Mick Fleetwood—member of Fleetwood Mac

Aretha Franklin—singer ("The Queen of Soul")

Melvin Franklin—member of The Temptations

Jerry Garcia—member of The Grateful Dead

Dizzy Gillespie—jazz musician

Shirley Horn—Grammy-winning jazz singer and pianist

Marvin Isley—member of The Isley Brothers

Mahalia Jackson—gospel singer

Randy Jackson—musician, producer, *American Idol* judge

Rick James—funk legend ("Super Freak")

Waylon Jennings—country singer

Nick Jonas—member of The Jonas Brothers

Herbert Kahury—musician ("Tiny Tim")

Ghostface Killah—member of Wu-Tang Clan

B.B. King—blues singer and musician

Patti LaBelle—soul singer

Peggy Lee—jazz singer (Grammy winner)

Tommy Lee—member of Motley Crüe

Meat Loaf—singer

Curtis Mayfield—soul singer

Bret Michaels—lead singer of Poison

Tim Parker—member of Blackalicious

James Phelps—gospel and rhythm and blues singer

Elvis Presley—musician ("The King Of Rock 'n' Roll")

Giacomo Puccini—operatic composer

Brenda Russell—singer-songwriter (Broadway's *The Color Purple*)

Sir Harry Secombe—Welsh singer, entertainer, former president of the British Diabetic Association

Angie Stone—singer

Jessica Stone—singer, actress

Elliott Yamin—singer, *American Idol* contestant

Neil Young—singer, songwriter, guitarist, and director

Gary Valenciano—Philippino singer

Luther Vandross—singer

Leslie West—guitarist, singer, songwriter

Norman Whitfield—rhythm and blues songwriter (Grammy winner), record producer

Brad Wilk—member of Rage Against the Machine, Audioslave

Scientists

Albert Ellis—pioneer of behavioral psychotherapy

Thomas Edison—inventor (light bulb, phonograph)

Cynthia Ice—IBM's Lotus accessibility lead and software developer

Dr. George Minot—first person with diabetes to receive Nobel Prize for Medicine

John Paul Stapp—doctor and space research pioneer, "The Fastest Man on Earth"

Movies About Diabetes

Diabetes has even made it into the movies. Although not all of these films were entirely realistic, uplifting, or focused primarily on diabetes, at the very least they created awareness. Let's get some more!

Alma (1997): Documentary film in which the main subject has diabetes.

Big Nothing (2006): Agent Hymes, nicknamed "The Eye," has diabetes, and the lead characters decide to kill him by forcing him to eat sugar until he dies. I have never even thought of being tortured that way. Wow, would that suck.

Bread & Roses (2000): Character Rosa is married to man who has diabetes, and they have financial hardship because of it. Of course, you can't live a normal life with diabetes, can you?

Brokedown Palace (1999): Father of main character Alice has diabetes.

Chocolat (2000): Judi Dench portrays a grandmother with diabetes. At the end, through the metaphor of chocolate, people are able to embrace a free lifestyle and sexual freedom and reject repression of all kinds. That wasn't available to the woman with diabetes, however. Dench's character dies of complications from diabetes presumably brought on by hanging out in the chocolate shop instead of adhering to a healthier diet.

Click (2006): Henry Winkler plays Ted, the father of Adam Sandler's main character Michael Newman. Ted has diabetes. I kind of like that the Fonz is on my side.

Con Air (1997): A prison parolee, played by Nicolas Cage, and another convict named Baby O whom he befriends are being transported on a maximum-security plane with some of the country's most dangerous criminals. After the plane is skyjacked, Baby O, who has diabetes, doesn't receive a scheduled insulin shot, and his syringes are destroyed during in-flight chaos. Moral of that story is to always pack extra supplies and keep them in your carry-on.

Derailed (2005): Lead male character's daughter has diabetes, and her third kidney transplant has failed.

Dog Day Afternoon (1975): The bank manager has diabetes.

It Runs in The Family (2003): Wife of Kirk Douglas character has diabetes and is on dialysis.

La Débandade (**a.k.a. *Hard Off***) (1999): Lead male character has diabetes.

Mad Money (2008): When character Jackie Truman (Katie Holmes) drops her purse, an insulin needle is among the items coworkers Bridget Cardigan (Diane Keaton) and Nina Brewster (Queen Latifah) help her to retrieve. Unaware of Jackie's diabetes, they assume she is a drug addict. Go-with-the-flow Jackie never corrects them, feeling that their show of concern makes the deception worthwhile.

Memento (2000): Main character's wife has diabetes. He kills her by giving her an overdose of insulin shots. This scares the crap out of me.

Nothing in Common (1986): Jackie Gleason portrays the father, a man who's estranged from his family while grappling with his diagnosis. He should have read this book.

Panic Room (2002): The young character, Sarah (Kristen Stewart), has diabetes and experiences an episode of low blood glucose (hypoglycemia) while trapped in the panic room with her mother.

Phonies Beware! (1956): Short film in which the Food and Drug Administration launches an investigation after a diabetes patient dies after using a drug claiming to be a cure for diseases such as diabetes.

Scarecrow Gone Wild (2004): Teen with diabetes goes into diabetic coma during a hazing incident and becomes a killer scarecrow. As though it isn't bad enough to be diabetic, you also have to become a crazed chunk of hay with a hankering for blood.

Soul Food (1997): Family matriarch Mamma Jo has diabetes.

Species (1995): Natasha Henstridge plays a half-human/half-alien creature who is grown on Earth but escapes and attempts to produce offspring with various men. She finds one man she thinks might be a potential mate, but kills him after she realizes he has a genetic flaw: diabetes. Heed the warning and stay away from aliens who are looking to mate with you.

Steel Magnolias (1989): Many moviegoers recall Julia Roberts in the movie with beads of sweat on her lip and brow, fighting an offer of orange juice from Sally Field during a severe hypoglycemic episode in Truvy's Salon. It was arguably the most famous scene depicting a person with diabetes in a major motion picture. I have actually seen people do this before. When your sugar is low, it's not time to argue. Drink the damn Kool-Aid.

The General (1998): The true story of Martin Cahill, a famous Irish gangster, played by Brendan Gleeson, who has type II diabetes.

The Godfather III (1990): Character Michael Corleone has diabetes.

The Next Three Days (2010): Russell Crowe plays John Brennan, a loyal husband and father desperate to free his wrongly imprisoned wife (played by Elizabeth Banks). She has diabetes, which plays a major role in his escape plan. My kind of movie. Use diabetes to your advantage.

The Witches (1990): The grandmother, Helga, is diagnosed with diabetes.

Warlock (1989): Character Kassandra is a person with type 1 diabetes. She uses a syringe in the end to help destroy the warlock. Sorry if I ruined the ending for you.

The above listings were originally compiled by dlist.com and edited by me for your reading pleasure.

Chapter Twelve

The Sugar-Coated Lining

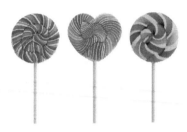

Do I ever get angry that I have diabetes? *Hell, yes!* I have the occasional moment. There is no one I can take it out on, no one to yell at, no one to punch, no one to blame. The big "D" is unpredictable, uncooperative, unforgiving, and relentless. So, our choices are to sit around feeling bad for ourselves or to use the disease to strengthen and empower us.

The odds of developing depression are greater in someone with diabetes than in someone without the disorder, and it's easy to slide down that slippery slope when the going gets tough. It has been proven that diabetes can cause depression because of the burden, guilt, anxiety, anger, hesitation, worry, fear, and embarrassment it can wreak on a person's psyche. It really can take its toll on a person's well-being. However, when you accept what you cannot change, and desire to live the best life possible, things get a lot easier. Happiness is a choice.

If I had to live the past twenty years over, I would have done things differently. Maybe I would have skipped college. My entrepreneurial spirit was well in place before my college years, so I know I would have still flourished, and I believe my diabetes would not have. If my immune system hadn't attacked itself, that diabetes cell would still be floating around unbroken and untriggered. Since there's nothing I can do about that now, I am working with what I've been given. I use my condition as a benchmark of comparison for all other challenges. If I can handle diabetes, I can handle anything that comes my way. So can you.

Diabetes has given me discipline, but it also has given me so much more than that. It has provided me with the knowledge and capability to educate and help other people with the disease. It has given me volunteering and fundraising opportunities as well as the potential to participate in medical trials and focus groups to help other people around the world. It is my bona fide calling to help the diabetic community.

Anyone who has tried to raise money for a cause knows it is no simple task, and asking someone for their firstborn seems like an easier feat than getting a $10 donation. The fact is, not many people care until they have someone very close to them affected, and by very close, I mean a child. Adults with diabetes are boring and hard to feel bad for. Only one out of four of my brothers has ever even contributed to my cause, and that's only because his awesome wife and I are very close, and she made it happen.

Trust me, I more than empathize with kids who have type 1 diabetes; it's terrible to have to deal with something like this at such a young age. I have the same illness they do, however, and it affects me in the same exact way. What is more important is that one day they will be my age and will, unfortunately, still have diabetes, and no one will care about them anymore either.

With social media, casting a fundraising net is a little easier but not a cakewalk. I've tried shock marketing to seek awareness and support: showing a picture of my hip covered in miniature bruises, sharing with people that I have taken more than 172,000 shots in my lifetime, informing friends how I had a scary low blood glucose of twenty last night and thought I was going to pass out. Many friends "Like" every other one of my social media status updates—except the updates that have anything to do with raising money for diabetes awareness. They pretend they never saw those. If I post a picture of my dog doing something amusing, however, I'll get thirty-six "Likes." That's not to say that I don't have some very loving and supportive people around me. I do. Besides my immediate family, I have loyal friends who always donate and are always there for me in times of diabetic need (They are also there with wine in hand on many nondiabetes-related occasions too.)

I also have friends who like to give me my shots whenever the opportunity arises, but I'm not so sure what to make of that one. Do they subconsciously want to hurt me, or is it just some sadistic personality disorder they have? Either way, I should start charging for it and donating the money to my cause.

I have supported JDRF since I was diagnosed. They are the leading global organization funding type 1 diabetes research. Their goal is to progressively remove the impact of type 1 diabetes from people's lives until we achieve a world without the disorder. I do the Walk to Cure Diabetes and participate in any other fundraising activities I can throughout the year.

The JDRF Walk to Cure Diabetes is always very emotional for me. I see all of these families wearing specially designed team T-shirts in support of the person for whom they are out there walking. There are thousands upon thousands of people banning together to help find a cure for exactly what I am fighting. We are all there to do our part, large or small. Someone they know personally is affected by it, but it all feels very intimate to me and very moving. I always start crying as the walk starts. I am even welling up with tears thinking about it now.

Along with JDRF, there are other organizations and charities making a huge difference. Among them are, The American Diabetes Association (ADA), Diabetes Research Institute, the Diabetes Research and Wellness Foundation and the Joslin Diabetes Center. I am proud to support and partner with any of them whenever I am able. There are countless opportunities for you to give back. Getting involved in fundraising events or volunteering is a great start.

As diabetics, we have heard about a cure for as long as we have had the disease. Researchers say it's coming, and I was told that promise the day I was diagnosed, twenty years ago. You might have heard of the islet cell transplant. Islet transplantation is the transfer of isolated islets from a donor pancreas into another person. Those islet cells then start to produce insulin, and the idea is that the person doesn't have to take insulin injections anymore. I ran to put myself on the list to get one. When I came up for review, I was dismissed rather quickly. It seems that the antirejection drugs you need to take for the rest of your life cause cancer, so the only people who were getting the transplant were those who had serious diabetic complications. Why would you risk a healthy diabetic person (what an oxymoron) with what is potentially behind curtain number one? Current data is also showing that the effects of the transplant disappear for over 50% of those treated after only one year. So, with the possibility of that cure off my list, I have my sights set on other therapies that hold significant promise:

The Artificial Pancreas

Also known as the bionic pancreas and making huge headlines lately, this series of increasingly sophisticated artificial pancreas systems eliminates blood glucose testing and automates delivery of insulin and additional hormones in the body.

Encapsulation

Implantable beta cell replacement therapies that restore insulin independence without the need for intensive immune suppression could have you live every day as if diabetes were not a part of your life.

Smart Insulin

This new form of insulin circulates in the bloodstream and turns on when it is needed and off when it's not. This could change our world and make life with diabetes so much easier.

Restoration

This is the biological cure for T1D. The body's beta cell function is restored, and the autoimmune attack is halted. Your pancreas is, once again, a working part of your anatomy. Welcome back! You've been missed dearly!

Prevention

Research is headed quickly in this direction, slowing or halting the progression of diabetes before insulin dependence develops, eliminating the risk of even developing the disease. To think that we could really have a world with type *none* is my wildest dream.

I have been a guinea pig in the name of science more than once—probably closer to six times. I just recently started a yearlong trial testing a faster-acting insulin. I hope I am part of the experimental group rather than the control group, because the idea of bringing down high blood sugars more quickly really excites me. The last time I participated in a new insulin study, I gained ten pounds. I lost it right after I finished the trial, but that best not happen again. See what I do for all of you?

I mentioned earlier that one of the things I love about having diabetes is being able to help other people with this condition. I am a life coach by occupation, and I cannot think of anything else I'd rather be doing. It's true that if you love what you are doing, it never seems like work. I coach people all over the world, with and without diabetes. Anyone looking to make a positive change in their life is my ideal client, whether they want to boost their confidence levels, find an inner passion, start a business, or lower their A1C levels. There is good reason my organization is called Be You Only Better. Everyone can take what they have been given, improve it, and become better. If you don't wake up every day better than you were yesterday, you need to focus on your life more.

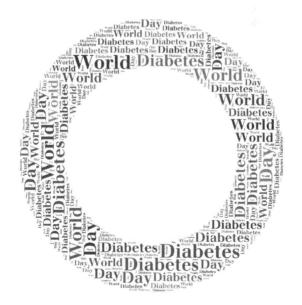

November is Diabetes Awareness Month, and it's a great time to focus on diabetes awareness. Many local schools, drugstores, and clinics hold free diabetes screenings, and you can have family members and other people whom you think might be affected checked out. November 14 has been declared World Diabetes Day by the United Nations, and the Blue Circle is now universally accepted as the symbol of diabetes awareness. Use it often. Weave it into your social media accounts. Get a T-shirt with it on the front. Wear it loud and proud. Organize events at a local school or arts center for students to design or decorate a blue circle to support the cause. Create events and have a portion of the ticket sales or entry fee or silent auction items go to benefit your charity of choice.

Don't be embarrassed by your disease. Stand up and be proud. Show the world that diabetes isn't controlling you. You are taking charge and controlling your diabetes. To do nothing is not an option. Whatever you do, the time and effort you spend will be greatly appreciated and rewarded.

Too often we get caught up in our own desires. We focus too much on ourselves and not enough on the needs of other people. By contributing to diabetes awareness you can focus on both. If you stop thinking about just yourself and concentrate on the contribution you're making to the rest of the world, you won't worry as much about your own issues but rather will see the big picture. This will increase self-confidence and allow you to contribute with maximum efficiency. The more you contribute to the world, the more you'll be rewarded with personal success and recognition. That goes the same whether you have diabetes or you don't.

Self-confidence is the difference between feeling unstoppable and feeling scared out of your wits. Your perception of yourself has an enormous impact on how others perceive you. Perception is reality; the more self-confidence you have, the more likely it is you'll succeed. Use your diabetes to bring you up, not push you down.

There are a number of things you can consciously do to build self-confidence and feel good about yourself. By applying the fifteen strategies below, you can get the mental edge you need to overcome any stigma you might think is attached to diabetes, bring happiness to your life, and reach your full potential. It's your time to SHINE!

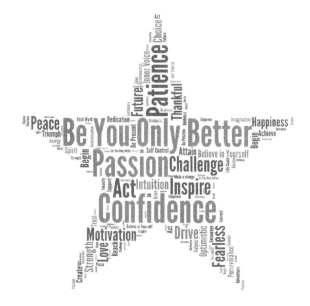

1. Do What You Love

Everyone loves to do something. When you indulge yourself in what you really enjoy, you improve the way you feel about yourself and improve your self-esteem while you are at it! Find your passion, and you find your purpose. Remember to make your own happiness a priority: your needs matter. If you do not value yourself, look out for yourself, and stick up for yourself, you are sabotaging yourself.

2. Help Others Out

Nothing makes you feel as warm and fuzzy as when you unselfishly care about and help others. Just do a good deed and lend a helping hand. It doesn't have to be big, and it doesn't have to cost any money. Learn compassion. Touch humanity. Help to ease the suffering of others. Even having a personal agenda like diabetes awareness still helps the world out as a whole when you volunteer your time and efforts. Love and kindness beget love and kindness.

3. Acknowledge Your Strengths

There is no one who has no strengths. Everyone is good at something. Know what you're good at, and share it with the world. Downplay your weaknesses. That's what all happy and successful people do. Never focus on them. Make a list to affirm to yourself all of your strengths, and then exercise them and give them more power. Be responsible for the talent that has been entrusted to you. In life it is rarely about getting a chance, it's about taking a chance. You are ready for that next step. Embrace opportunities and accept the challenges.

4. Face Your Fears

What are you most afraid of? What is holding you back? Whatever it might be, identify it and face it. Having experiences that make you face your fear is what really builds self-confidence. There is no way around it. Running away from your fears doesn't make them go away; it just makes them bigger than ever. Get them out in the open. What is it that scares you so much? Examine exactly what it is. Be honest with yourself as well. Trying to convince yourself they're not there doesn't make them go away. Next, educate yourself on your fears. Before you can face them, you need to learn more about what makes you fearful of these situations. It could be from a past experience, something that has caused you to never forget and has made you fearful since. It could also be from hearing someone else speak about a situation or even from watching it on TV. It's important to educate yourself on all the facts that make you fearful of this situation and start to give yourself the courage to face them. Once you do what it is that scares you most, you will feel strong, empowered, and fearless when you are done!

5. Lose Your Negative Friends

Hang out with people who are positive and support you and bring you up. It may be fun to have a bitchfest with friends occasionally, but if you hang out with these types of people too often, you will eventually become one of them. Those people are never happy. Life is too short to spend time with people who suck the happiness out of you. You will encounter many unenlightened folks when it comes time to your diabetes. Don't let them get to you. Instead, spend time with the people you enjoy, people who love and appreciate you and encourage you to improve in healthy and exciting ways. These people embrace who you are now so you can grow and embody who you want to be, unconditionally.

6. Pay Attention to Body Language

One of the easiest ways to tell how a person feels about herself is to examine her walk. Is it slow? Tired? Painful? Or is it energetic and purposeful? People with confidence walk quickly and with their head up and their eyes focused. They have places to go and people to see. Even if you aren't in a hurry, you can increase your self-confidence by having a skip in your step. Walking just a little faster will make you look and feel more important. Similarly, the way a person carries himself tells a story. People with slumped shoulders and lethargic movements display a lack of self-confidence. They aren't enthusiastic about what they're doing, and they don't consider themselves important. By practicing good posture, you'll automatically feel more confident. Stand up straight, keep your head up, and make eye contact. You'll make a positive impression on others and instantly feel more alert and empowered.

7. Value the Lessons Your Mistakes Teach You

Mistakes are okay; they are the stepping stones of progress. Take full accountability for your own life. You are the only one who can control the direction of your life. The extent to which you achieve your dreams depends on the extent to which you take responsibility for your own life. When you blame others for what you are going through, you deny responsibility and give others power over that part of your life. If you are not failing from time to time, you're not trying hard enough and you're not learning. Take risks, stumble, fall, and then get up and try again. Appreciate that you are pushing yourself, learning, growing, and improving. Significant achievements are almost invariably realized at the end of a long road of failures. One of the "mistakes" you fear might just be the link to your greatest achievement yet.

8. Live in the Moment

We hear this so often, but what does it really mean? Instead of waiting for the big things to happen—marriage, a promotion, the birth of a child—find joy in the smaller things that happen every day. Little things like staring up into a blue sky, a quiet cup of coffee in the morning, the smell of homemade cookies fresh from the oven, or the feel of warm rain on your face. Take notice of the world. Try to take notice of one particular sense and block out the others. Feel the environment around you. Feel the humidity in the air, the slant of the sun's warmth, or the briskness of wind through your hair. Fill your lungs with the scents of the day—pleasant aromas, sharp odors, fresh cut grass, and even sensory hints that are barely there, like soap lingering in the shower. Noticing these small pleasures on a daily basis make a big difference. Living in the moment means tuning into your senses and focusing on what you are doing right now. Slow down. Pause. Take the world in.

9. Practice Gratitude

When you focus too much on what you want, the mind creates reasons why you can't have it. This leads you to dwell on your weaknesses. The best way to avoid this is consciously focusing on gratitude. Set aside time each day to mentally list everything you have to be grateful for. Recall your past successes, unique skills, loving relationships, and positive momentum. Remain conscious of your blessings and victories. You'll be amazed how much you have going for you and be motivated to take that next step toward success. Look for the silver lining in tough situations. Remind yourself that you can and will grow stronger from whatever it is you are going through. Diabetes is a perfect example of that. Wake up and smile and set the tone of your entire day that way. Each new day is a gift. Treat it as such.

10. Compliment Other People

When we think negatively about ourselves, we often project that feeling onto others as insults and gossip. To break this cycle of negativity, get in the habit of praising other people. Be happy for those making progress. Look at yourself the same way. Compliment yourself on your great day of blood sugars or on how many times you tested. Celebrate the small victories. By looking for the best in others, you indirectly bring out the best in yourself. While you are complimenting other people, you also need to receive compliments with grace. It's hard to accept a compliment and easy to dismiss it by putting yourself down. For instance, when someone tells says you look great, you respond, "Really, that's hard to believe, I had no sleep last night," or if your friend tells you that you look like you lost weight, you might think, "Why, was I fat before?" A simple thank you is all that is needed.

11. Sit in the Front Row

In schools, offices, and public assemblies around the world, people constantly strive to sit at the back of the room. Most people prefer the back because they're afraid of being noticed. This reflects a lack of self-confidence. By deciding to sit in the front row, you can get over this irrational fear and build your self-confidence. You'll be more visible to the important people talking and from the front of the room, and you will learn more. Race for those front-row spots like you would at a U2 concert (or One Direction, depending on how old you are). Let that be symbolic for anything you do in life.

12. Speak Up

During group discussions many people never speak up because they're afraid that people will judge them for saying something stupid. This fear isn't really justified. People are generally much more accepting than we imagine. In fact, most people are dealing with the exact same fears. By making an effort to speak up at least once in every group discussion, you'll become a better public speaker, more confident in your own thoughts, and recognized as a leader by your peers. Diabetes is a great example of a subject you probably know a lot about and can speak up about often.

13. Work Out

Just as personal appearance affects confidence levels, so does physical fitness. If you're out of shape, you'll feel insecure, unattractive, and less energetic. By working out, you improve your physical appearance, energize yourself, and accomplish something positive. Having the discipline to work out not only makes you feel better, but it also creates positive momentum on which you can build for the rest of the day. You will feel more alive, and your blood glucose levels will improve!

14. Include Positivity in Your Life

Look at the positive angle for everything. Eliminate the self-doubt and the negative talk and replace them with positive thoughts and solutions. The mind must believe it *can* do something before it is actually capable of doing it. The way to overcome negative thoughts and destructive emotions is to develop opposing positive emotions that are stronger and more powerful. Regardless of the situation, focus on how you want it to turn out and what you want to happen and then take the next positive step forward. Just because you had a day of bad blood sugars does not make you a bad diabetic. Maybe your blood sugar wasn't great that day, but you exercised, or made an effort to count carbs. Focus on the little victories and where you want to be and follow the path to getting there.

15. Make No Comparisons

You absolutely cannot, under any circumstances, compare yourself with someone else. There is always going to be someone prettier, richer, skinnier, more successful, and not living with diabetes every day. Be inspired by, appreciate, and learn from others, but understand that competing against them is a waste of time. Just compare yourself with the self that you were yesterday. If you see improvement, great. If not, you have something to work on. Aim to break your own personal records.

Remember that confidence is all. The more confidence you have in yourself and belief that diabetes doesn't control you, you control it, the more successful you will be in every endeavor and the happier you will be in life! Awake every morning, test your blood sugar, trust that today is going to be the best day of your life, and watch how your world changes

Chapter Thirteen

Diabetic Lingo

This glossary is chock full of diabetes-related words (many completely made up) for easy reference and to spice up your diabetic vocabulary.

A1C test: A blood test that gauges how well you're managing your diabetes by reflecting your average blood sugar level for the past two to three months. Having a level under 7 percent indicates you are doing a good job and minimizes your risk of future complications. Keep in mind that the lower the A1C, the greater the hypoglycemia risk, so don't go striving for under 6 percent.

B12 shots: The Wonder Woman / Superman shot. Improves energy, boosts mood and the immune system, slows aging, and helps you to leap tall buildings in a single bound.

BG: Lazy term for blood glucose used when writing it over and over in a book.

The big D: Self-explanatory.

Bitch: Female dog or the word I have used multiple times to describe people who are insensitive toward diabetes and those with the disorder.

Bolus worthy: Something really yummy that you know will raise your blood sugar but is worth eating.

Bouncing: When your blood sugar drops so low in the middle of the night that your liver kicks in some glucose, causing you to bounce from low to high and usually back again. (See also *Roller-coastering*.)

Blood glucose monitor: Next to insulin this is your life line. A requirement for those with diabetes.

Bloody constellation: When you prick your finger and squeeze it and about five holes show up with blood, closely resembling the Big Dipper.

Born-again diabetic: A person with diabetes who has a newfound interest in taking care of him- or herself after years of negligence and denial. Welcome back to the club!

Candy drawer: Where all the guilty pleasures are and the first place you go when you have a low. When the candy drawer is empty of your hypo-stash and *you* didn't empty it, nondiabetics nearby had better watch their backs.

Carbonese: The language of carbohydrate counting.

Carbs: Evil, organic compounds that your body uses to make glucose and that you need insulin to combat.

Continuous glucose monitor: A handy-dandy tiny sensor inserted under the skin to check glucose levels in tissue. Fancier but not as accurate as a standard glucose meter.

Crashing: When blood sugar drops low and fast. This can sometimes result from a *rage bolus.*

D-day: The day you were diagnosed. You should try to get yourself a present on that day. Even better, have other people get you presents.

Darting: Injecting and testing. Needles going in and out of your skin multiple times daily.

Dawn phenomenon: An early morning increase in blood sugar that doesn't result from ingesting carbs.

Daylight Saving Time: Time to change the lancet.

Dead strips: Used glucose strips found in random spots: in the cup holder of your car, in your bed, in your dog's mouth.

Di-ah-bee-tis: The annoying way the old guy on the commercial pronounces diabetes. Like nails on a chalkboard to us diabetics.

Diabetes mellitus: The official name for this fabulous disease, derived from the Greek word for *siphon or flowing* (diabetes) and the Latin word for *sweet honey* (mellitus).

Diabetic PMS: When blood sugar skyrockets for no apparent reason in the two or three days prior to the start of a woman's cycle.

Dia-badass: Everyone living with the disease who doesn't let it push them around.

Diabulimia: Using high blood sugars to produce ketones and, in turn, lose weight. This is extremely dangerous and not a joking matter.

Dry spiking: Taking repeated blood sugar tests, but no blood wants to come out.

Gestational diabetes: The diabetes you might get when you are preggo. Type 1 and type 2 diabetics are excluded.

Gusher: When you prick your finger and are assaulted by your own bloodstream. Also sometimes found when you remove an infusion site.

Highway checks: When the person with diabetes juggles the steering wheel, blood glucose meter, test strips, lancet, and target finger. Commonly occurs in the dark.

Honeymoon phase: Equivalent to a remission. Some of the insulin-producing beta cells of the pancreas haven't been completely destroyed yet and produce unpredictable amounts of insulin, making you believe perhaps you have been cured.

Hooking: When your pump tubing snags the doorknob and almost rips out your internal organs along with your infusion set. Almost always results in shouting a profanity. (See also *Pump lassoing*.)

Hypoglycemia: Low blood sugar. Time to indulge your sweet tooth.

Hyperglycemia: High blood sugar. Bring on the insulin.

Instinctual bolus: Taking more insulin that your carbonese skills deem necessary because you "know" you are going to go high.

Insulin balls: Hard orbs of insulin beneath the skin that result from a poorly absorbed insulin injection. Often take hours to disappear and leave a black and blue mark in their wake.

Insulin pump: A small, computerized piece of technology that delivers insulin at a continuous dose (basal) and at your direction (bolus). Has revolutionized the management of diabetes.

Juvenile diabetes: An antiquated term that we now refer to as type 1 diabetes. Much like Trix cereal, "It's not just for kids!"

Ketones: A chemical produced when there is a shortage of insulin in the blood, and the body breaks down body fat for energy. It's a sign that your body is using fat for energy instead of using glucose because not enough insulin is available to use glucose for energy. Super dangerous to those with diabetes.

Live-abetes: The opposite of diabetes. We live life fully with this disease every day!

Neuropathy: Damage to the nerves in the peripheral nervous system. You don't want this.

Pancreas: Lazy son of a bitch.

Poker: That thing that you put your lancet in to check your blood sugar.

Prediabetes: You'd better start taking care of yourself pronto, or we will regretfully welcome you to the type 2 club.

Prickupine: An imaginary animal you most resemble after jabbing yourself way too many times in a short window of time.

Pump lassoing: Accidentally snagging your tubing around something (like a knob on a drawer) and either pulling your setting from your body or coming dangerous close to it. (See also *Hooking.*)

Rapid checker: The use of more than five test strips in less than an hour because you are not sure which way your blood sugar is going.

Rage bolus: Taking repeated doses of insulin when your sugar won't come down, knowing full well you will end up with a low later.

Retinopathy: Acute damage to the retina. You definitely don't want this.

Roller-coastering: High blood sugar followed by a low blood sugar followed by a high blood sugar followed by a low blood sugar. (See also *Bouncing.*)

Scarlet D: The red letter you might as well go around wearing that lets the world know you have diabetes.

Sleepeating: The act of waking in the middle of the night, going to the kitchen, and eating anything you can find when you have a low.

The sugar: Slang name for diabetes that originates from the South. We like our tea sweet and our diabetics sweeter.

Sugar reaper: A nighttime hypoglycemia that nearly kills you.

Type 1 diabetes: The autoimmune disease in which a person's pancreas stops producing insulin, a hormone that enables people to get energy from food. It usually strikes in childhood or young adulthood and lasts a lifetime, causing type 1 diabetics to take multiple injections of insulin daily or continually infuse through a pump.

Type 2 diabetes: A metabolic disorder in which a person's body still produces insulin but cannot use it effectively. It is often diagnosed in adulthood and does not always require insulin.

Type 3 diabetic: A person who is "diabetic by association." Can be a parent, spouse, child, friend, or anyone close enough to you who truly understands what diabetes is all about. Often the fetcher of something sweet and usually subject to low blood sugar rants.

The End

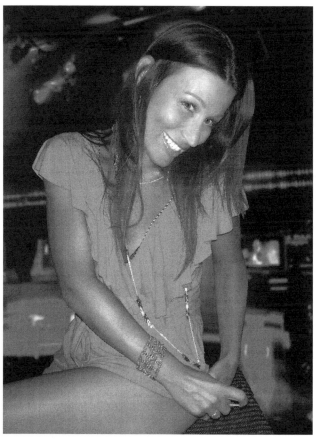

*Diabetes doesn't always have to be
a pain in the ass.*

21446771R00102

Made in the USA
Middletown, DE
30 June 2015